50 Foot Challenges –
ASSESSMENT AND MANAGEMENT

Colin E. Thomson BSc(Hons) FCPod(S)

Lecturer, Queen Margaret University College,
Edinburgh; Associate Clinician, The Royal Infirmary
of Edinburgh, Edinburgh, UK

J. N. Alastair Gibson MD FRCS(Orth)

Consultant Trauma and Orthopaedic Surgeon,
The Royal Infirmary of Edinburgh; Part-time Senior
Lecturer, The University of Edinburgh, Edinburgh, UK

Foreword by

Geoffrey Hooper FRCSEd(Orth)

Consultant Orthopaedic Surgeon, St John's Hospital,
Livingston, West Lothian, UK

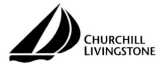
CHURCHILL LIVINGSTONE

EDINBURGH LONDON NEW YORK OXFORD PHILADELPHIA ST LOUIS SYDNEY
TORONTO 2002

CHURCHILL LIVINGSTONE
An imprint of Elsevier Science Limited

First published 2002
Reprinted 2003

ISBN 0 443 06495 4

British Library Cataloguing in Publication Data
A catalogue record for this book is available from the British Library.

Library of Congress Cataloging in Publication Data
A catalog record for this book is available from the Library of Congress.

Note
Medical knowledge is constantly changing. As new information becomes available, changes in treatment, procedures, equipment and the use of drugs become necessary. The authors and the publishers have taken care to ensure that the information given in this text is accurate and up to date. However, readers are strongly advised to confirm that the information, especially with regard to drug usage, complies with the latest legislation and standards of practice.

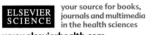

ELSEVIER
SCIENCE
your source for books,
journals and multimedia
in the health sciences

www.elsevierhealth.com

The
publisher's
policy is to use
paper manufactured
from sustainable forests

Printed in China
C/02

50 Foot Challenges –
Assessment and Management

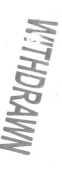

To
Eilidh and Mhairi
Arran, Rory and Caitlin

For Churchill Livingstone:

Editorial Director, Health Professions: Mary Law
Project Development Manager: Dinah Thom
Project Manager: Andrea Hill
Designer: Judith Wright
Illustrations: Judith Watson

CONTENTS

FOREWORD

This book takes a novel approach to foot disorders. The two authors, one a podiatrist and the other an orthopaedic surgeon, guide us through the diagnosis and management of some common (and some not so common) disorders, using illustrated case histories. This practical approach is akin to taking part in a teaching session in the outpatient clinic, and is much more realistic than reading abstract descriptions in a textbook. Those learning about foot disorders for the first time will pick up a lot of valuable information, and more experienced practitioners will also find a great deal to interest them.

Foot disorders are responsible for a great deal of misery, and anything that helps to improve the diagnosis of common foot conditions and their correct treatment is to be welcomed. I enjoyed reading this book and I am sure that you will too.

Geoffrey Hooper

PREFACE

In compiling this book it has been our aim to provide a self-assessment text that allows readers to test their knowledge on a wide variety of conditions of the foot, some common, some less so. It has not been our ambition to write a comprehensive reference text on the foot; for this purpose there are already many excellent texts. Instead we have tried to make available useful information in a concise and accessible format that is easy to read and user-friendly, with a prominent pictorial content.

We offer you 50 cases that we hope will present a series of challenges to all those involved in treating the foot. We have set the reader problems of varying difficulty, the solutions for which are suggested on the subsequent pages with an expanded discussion of the condition in question. Key references are listed as well as summary points. We have included, where appropriate, 'clinical tips' which will aid your practice.

It is not essential to use this book as a self-assessment text, as it will serve equally well as a short guide to a broad range of foot conditions. For your convenience we have grouped these conditions into seven sections.

We hope that by the end of this text you will have graduated to become a 'foot expert'.

Edinburgh 2002

Colin E. Thomson
J. N. Alastair Gibson

ACKNOWLEDGEMENTS

We are indebted to Mr Mike Devlin of the Department of Clinical Photography at the Royal Infirmary of Edinburgh, who has expertly taken many of the clinical photographs printed in the book. We also thank Judith Watson for her drawings and our colleagues Malcolm Macnicol (Figs 21.1–3), John McGregor (Fig. 27.2) and Donald Salter (Fig. 30.2) for providing clinical slides.

Figures 14.1, 14.2 and 18.1 are reproduced by permission of Churchill Livingstone from Wilkinson J D & Shaw S 1998 Colour Guide Dermatology; Figure 17.2 is reproduced by permission of Churchill Livingstone from Gawkrodger D J 2000 Dermatology, An Illustrated Colour Text; Figures 20.2, 35.2 and 37.4 are reproduced by permission of Churchill Livingstone from Moll J M H 1997 Colour Guide Rheumatology; Figure 36.2 is reproduced by permission of Mosby-Wolfe from Jones W A & Owen R 1995 A Colour Atlas of Clinical Orthopaedics; Figure 41.1 is reproduced by permission of Churchill Livingstone from Krentz A J 1997 Colour Guide Diabetes.

ABBREVIATIONS

ABPI	Ankle:brachial pressure index
AP	Anteroposterior
DIP	Distal interphalangeal
IP	Interphalangeal
MRI	Magnetic resonance image
MTP	Metatarsophalangeal
PIP	Proximal interphalangeal
RA	Rheumatoid arthritis
SACH	Solid ankle cushion heel

Orthopaedics

ORTHOPAEDICS

CASE 1

A 45-year-old ex-ballerina presents with a painful great toe and dorsal swelling as shown in Figure 1.1.

1. This patient had virtually no movement at her metatarsophalangeal (MTP) joint. What terms are used to describe restricted movement at the first MTP joint?

2. Young patients with this condition often report that they have participated in competitive sport. Which sports are particularly bad for your toe and what other conditions will lead to the radiographic appearances shown in Figure 1.2?

3. What anatomical variations may predispose a patient to hallux rigidus?

4. What modifications to the patient's shoes might lessen her pain?

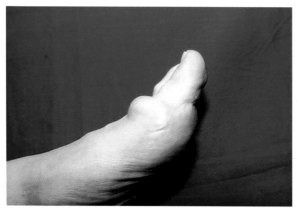

Fig. 1.1 Dorsal bunion overlying hallux MTP joint

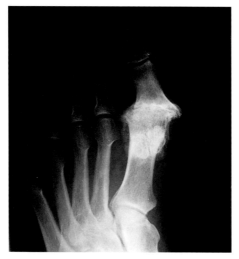

Fig. 1.2 Radiograph of great toe

Aetiology of hallux rigidus

1. The dorsal prominence seen is indicative of underlying degenerative osteoarthritis and dorsal osteophyte formation. Limitation and absence of movement are termed hallux 'limitus' and 'rigidus', respectively.

2. Degenerative joint arthritis arises from direct cartilage damage, and players of any sport who kick a ball repetitively are prone to hallux rigidus. In American footballers the condition is labelled 'turf toe'. Sepsis, inflammatory arthritis or excessive repetitive weight transfer (a similar factor to that causing osteochondritis of the second metatarsal head), all potentially lead to the same end result.

3. Several factors have been described that may contribute to the development of hallux rigidus. Elongation of the first metatarsal, or its dorsiflexion, will alter not only the pattern of stress placed across the forefoot, but will also change the dynamics of the articulation between the sesamoids and the first metatarsal head. Clearly, pronation of the forefoot leading to pes planus will also contribute to excessive joint wear.

4. Two factors produce symptoms and it may be important to address one or both of these. Firstly, as osteoarthritis of the MTP joint progresses, the joint space narrows which leads to tendon and ligament contractures and associated stiffness. Secondly, osteophytes form around the margins of the joint, particularly dorsally and laterally, leading to a mechanical block to extension and sometimes hallux flexus.

Transient benefits may be gained from simple conservative treatments. Non-steroidal anti-inflammatory drugs, rest and elevation of the foot may all help if the toe is particularly sore. The authors have not found that intra-articular steroid injections provide anything other than short-term pain relief, but a rigid insole should restrict joint movement sufficiently to lessen pain (Fig. 1.3). A rocker bar on the sole is also worth fitting as this acts to offload the first metatarsal head by reducing the need for joint extension at 'toe-off' (Fig. 1.4).

If these treatments fail, then patients will generally consider surgery.

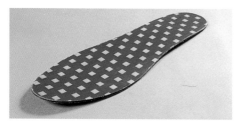

Fig. 1.3 Carbonflex insole

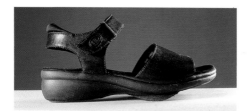

Fig. 1.4 Rocker sole

KEY POINTS

- Hallux rigidus is a degenerative condition.
- Painful joint extension prevents normal gait.
- A rocker bar fitted to the shoe sole may be helpful.

FURTHER READING

Horton GA, Park Y-W, Myerson MS (1999) Role of metatarsus primus elevatus in the pathogenesis of hallux rigidus. Foot and Ankle International 20:777–80.

Smith RW, Katchis SD, Ayson LC (2000) Outcomes in hallux rigidus patients treated nonoperatively: a long-term follow-up study. Foot and Ankle International 21:906–13.

CASE 2

A distinctive bony prominence has developed overlying this lady's second metatarsal head (Fig. 2.1). She is 61 years old, retired and has a long-standing history of pain in her right foot. On examination, movement at her MTP joint was severely restricted.

1. Given the objective symptoms, explain the presence of this dorsal prominence.

2. Describe the pathology of the condition.

3. Do conservative measures have anything to offer this patient?

4. What are the surgical options?

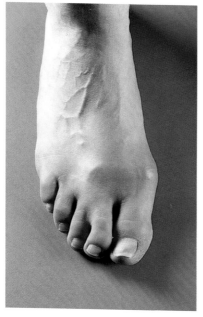

Fig. 2.1 Clinical appearance of the foot showing distinctive dorsal prominence

Freiberg's infraction

1. Osteochondritis of the second metatarsal head, termed Freiberg's infraction, is a common, crushing-type osteochondritis leading to avascular necrosis. It most commonly arises in adolescent girls but may also affect boys. Although this patient does remember an episode of a painful foot as a youngster, she did not present until later life when she developed pain in her second MTP joint.

2. The head of the metatarsal progressively collapses or 'infracts' into the avascular segment (Fig. 2.2). This leads to flattening of the metatarsal articular surface, head compression and loss of joint space. The later changes are those of secondary osteoarthritis (Fig. 2.3).

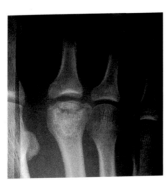

Fig. 2.2 AP radiograph: infraction of second metatarsal head

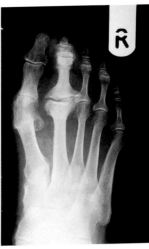

Fig. 2.3 AP radiograph: osteoarthritis of second MTP joint

3. Adaptations to footwear, namely a rocker sole, may be advantageous as they aid dorsiflexion of the foot. Local injections of hydrocortisone provide only short-term symptomatic relief.

4. In the older patient, where degenerative changes are the cause of discomfort, either a proximal hemiphalangectomy or, as in this case, a joint replacement arthroplasty will be required (Fig. 2.4). In younger patients, Gauthier's procedure restores joint congruity by rotating the 'normal' dorsal cartilage onto the articulating surface (Fig. 2.5a and b).

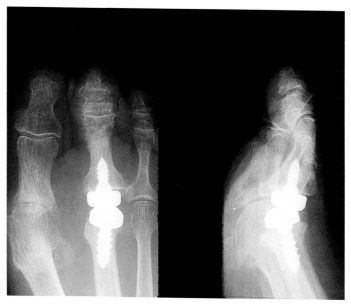

Fig. 2.4 AP and lateral radiographs showing replacement arthroplasty of the second MTP joint

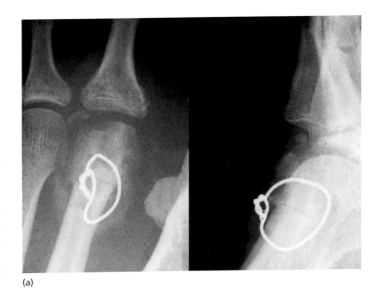

(a)

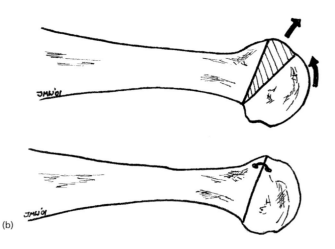

(b)

Fig. 2.5 (a) AP and lateral radiograph of Gauthier's procedure and (b) illustration of Gauthier's procedure (lateral view)

KEY POINTS

- Freiberg's infraction is a disease of adolescence.
- The condition is an avascular necrosis of the metatarsal head.
- Secondary osteoarthritis always develops.
- In older patients, replacement or resection arthroplasty may be necessary.

FURTHER READING

Hay SM, Smith TWD (1992) Freiberg's disease: an unusual presentation at the age of 50 years. The Foot 2:176–8.

Smith TWD, Stanley D, Rowley DI (1991) Treatment of Freiberg's disease: a new operative technique. Journal of Bone and Joint Surgery 73-B:129–30.

CASE 3

A middle-aged lady complains of a painful second toe when walking. Her shoe has rubbed on the toe for some years.

1. Which digital deformity is this and what causes it?

2. What treatment options are there?

3. Is there any specific therapy that might prevent the deformity recurring following surgery?

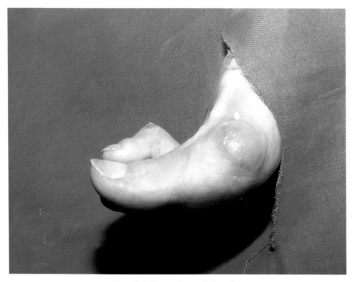

Fig. 3.1 Second toe deformity

Hammer toe

1. The photograph shows the typical appearance of hammering of the second toe (Fig. 3.1). This condition is distinguishable from claw toe (Fig. 3.2) in which there is greater flexion of the distal interphalangeal (IP) joint and dorsal subluxation of the MTP joint. In mallet toe the distal IP joint only is flexed (Fig. 3.3).

Hammer toe is often familial and usually gradually progressive from a young age. Frequently the second toe and/or the second metatarsal is abnormally long: i.e. the foot is 'index minus' or of 'Greek' type, respectively, and such a deformity leads to increased tension, at least on the medial aspect of the plantar aponeurosis. Direct pull onto the plantar plate and flexor tendon sheath at the level of the MTP joint explains the joint flexion. In the elderly, since the aponeurosis stretches out with age, there does have to be some dorsiflexion of the proximal phalanx before flexion of the proximal interphalangeal (PIP) joint will occur.

2. PIP joint fusion is probably the most commonly performed surgical procedure for hammer toe. Resection of the joint produces a relative lengthening of the dorsal extensor

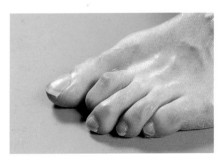

Fig. 3.2 Claw toe

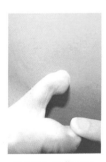

Fig. 3.3 Mallet toe

tendon. This may be sufficient to prevent subluxation of the proximal phalanx dorsally on the metatarsal. If not, it is worthwhile performing a dorsal capsulotomy of the MTP joint and possibly also a transfer of the dorsal extensor tendon to the metatarsal head. Flexor to extensor transfer will not provide sufficient pull in an adult to correct the deformity.

Hohman recommended excision of the head of the proximal phalanx and reefing of the dorsal extensor tendon. The authors have generally found that this produces an inferior result to fusion, as some patients will experience continuing discomfort from the mobile joint. We would not recommend either proximal hemiphalangectomy (Fig. 3.4), which may leave a redundant and shortened digit, or amputation (Fig. 3.5).

3. After PIP joint arthrodesis it is worthwhile prescribing a metatarsal dome insole to support the second metatarsal head (Fig. 3.6).

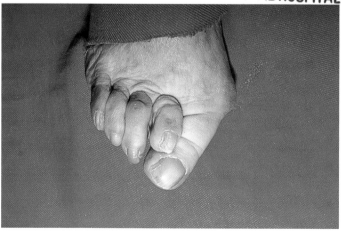

Fig. 3.4 Appearance after proximal hemiphalangectomy

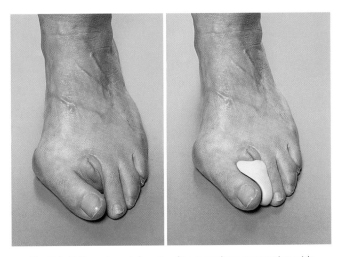

Fig. 3.5 Hallux valgus deformity after second toe amputation with and without spacer

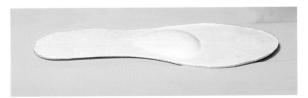

Fig. 3.6 Metatarsal dome support

KEY POINTS

- Dorsal and terminal corns will arise secondary to fixed flexion of the PIP toe joint.
- Operative treatment is generally beneficial.
- PIP joint fusion is probably the commonest procedure performed.
- A metatarsal dome support may be helpful.

FURTHER READING

American College of Foot and Ankle Surgeons (1999) Hammer toe syndrome. Journal of Foot and Ankle Surgery 38:166–78.

Harmonson JK, Harkless LB (1996) Operative procedures for the correction of hammer toe, claw toe, and mallet toe: a literature review. Clinics in Podiatric Medicine and Surgery 13:211–20.

CASE 4

A 76-year-old ex-army major presented with a request for new shoes. He stated that his feet had always been broad and that they had not inhibited his military service (Fig. 4.1).

Earlier in the same clinic a 45-year-old patient had presented with a similarly broad foot (Fig. 4.2).

1. What is the aetiology of polydactyly and is there a common pattern?

2. How will treatment vary for the different types of anomaly?

3. Would there be any indication for surgery in this elderly man?

4. What term is used to describe the enlarged toe shown in Figure 4.2 and what treatment options might be considered?

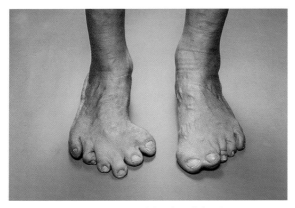

Fig. 4.1 Congenital forefoot deformity

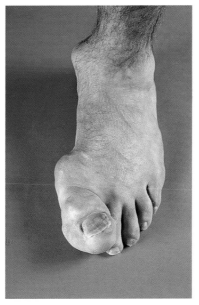

Fig. 4.2 Great toe hypertrophy

Polydactyly and macrodactyly

1. The slide shows polydactyly. This condition occurs most frequently as a result of duplication of the fifth toe (up to 80%) or, as in this case, of the first ray. Middle toe duplication is much less common. The duplication may involve any part of the involved digit, or the metatarsal. In this case the phalanges were duplex (Fig. 4.3).

2. Treatment of polydactyly is generally straightforward. The smallest digit, which may well be rudimentary, should be excised and the skin carefully closed by direct suture or rotational flaps as necessary. Preaxial (hallux) duplication may be associated with hallux varus and this problem must be addressed separately.

3. This elderly gentleman had never suffered any impairment of foot function as a result of his broad forefeet. Indeed, he had served in the army throughout the war, passing all the

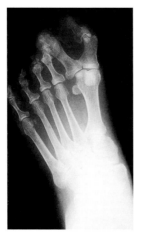

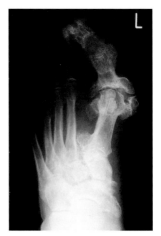

Fig. 4.3 Polydactyly: AP radiograph of left foot

Fig. 4.4 Gigantism: AP radiograph showing widening of the first ray

fitness tests. There would be absolutely no indication now to offer any form of treatment other than custom footwear.

4. Metatarsal or phalangeal duplication may lead to gigantism, but more commonly an entire ray is enlarged (Fig. 4.4).

The soft tissue swelling observed was typical of that seen in both classical gigantism caused by neurofibromatosis and in association with hyperdynamic circulation arising from arteriovenous malformations. In fact, in this case there was evidence of excess fat deposition within the marrow and the patient was diagnosed as suffering from macrodystrophia lipomatosa. The disproportionate increase in fibroadipose tissue is a form of hamartoma.

KEY POINTS

- Postaxial polydactyly is most common.
- Indications for surgery may be functional or cosmetic.
- The least functional digit should be excised.
- Digital gigantism may occur in association with neurofibromatosis.

FURTHER READING

Phelps DA, Grogan DP (1985) Polydactyly of the foot. Journal of Pediatric Orthopaedics 5:446–51.

Shaheed N, Nealy JA, Bituin BV (2000) A rare occurrence of polydactyly. Journal of the American Podiatric Medicine Association 90:425–9.

Sobel E, Giorgini RJ, Potter GK, Schwartz RD, Chieco TM (2000) Progressive pedal macrodactyly surgical history with 15 year follow-up. Foot and Ankle International 21:45–50.

CASE 5

A 66-year-old woman presents with a tender bunion. Examination reveals a large bursal swelling and some hammering of the lesser digits (Figs 5.1 and 5.2). She stated that the bunion had progressively enlarged over a few years.

1. What is the probable underlying cause of this lady's hallux valgus?

2. What factors have led to the hammering of this lady's lesser toes? If the second digit had been overriding, might amputation have been worthwhile?

3. In this case the patient had just recovered from a heart attack and did not wish to consider any form of surgery. What conservative measures might help to relieve her discomfort?

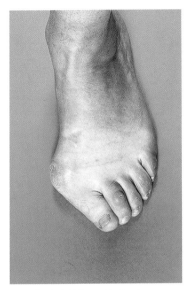

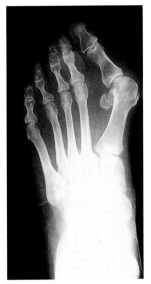

Fig. 5.1 Enlarged hallux bursa

Fig. 5.2 Standing AP radiograph

Aetiology of hallux valgus

1. Many factors have been considered to be causative of hallux valgus. Probably the least important of these is the 'wearing of tight fitting shoes'. Foot pronation, together with metatarsus primus varus, is generally evident in most patients presenting with 'bunions'. Lesser factors almost certainly include an abnormally acute cuneiform/first metatarsal angle and an insufficiency of the intermetatarsal band between the first and second metatarsal heads.

Once the hallux has deviated laterally, the medial capsule of the MTP joint will be stretched and the sesamoids pulled laterally away from their normal plantar articulation on the underside of the first metatarsal head. The hallux deviation will be accentuated by the pull of the long flexor and extensor tendons, and the joint reaction forces created serve to push the metatarsal head even further medially.

2. In most instances hammering of a digit can be traced to a relative discrepancy in the length of the adjacent digits. It is particularly relevant if the patient has a 'Greek' type foot with an excessively long second metatarsal.

Amputation is contraindicated even if the second toe is overriding the hallux. Removal of the second toe serves only to accentuate any hallux valgus and allows the sesamoids to displace even further laterally. The patient would then tend to offload the first ray by taking more weight on the lateral side of her foot.

3. Many elderly patients have lived with their foot deformities for many years. It is essential to provide comfortable shoes and these must usually be made to measure. A toe box with sufficient depth to accommodate the overriding digits is required.

KEY POINTS

- Surgery for hallux valgus is rarely obligatory.
- Wide fitting shoes with sufficient room to accommodate the toes may be all that is required.
- Digit realignment generally requires metatarsal osteotomy.

FURTHER READING

Bryant A, Tinley P, Singer K (2000) A comparison of radiographic measurements in normal, hallux valgus, and hallux limitus feet. Journal of Foot and Ankle Surgery 39:39–43.

CASE 6

Runners can be plagued with a number of foot problems and the condition described here is particularly annoying. Left heel pain has troubled this 32-year-old male long distance runner for some months. He reports no specific injury and describes his pain as sharp and usually worse first thing in the morning. With exercise his pain diminishes, then recurs after rest. Examination reveals tenderness in the centre of his heel pad (Fig. 6.1) and a lateral radiograph is shown (Fig. 6.2).

1. Given the presenting symptoms, what is the most likely cause of this athlete's pain?

2. Why is pain worse first thing in the morning?

3. Describe the examination taking place in Figure 6.1.

4. What is shown in the X-ray in Figure 6.2 and what is its significance?

5. Outline a treatment plan for this patient.

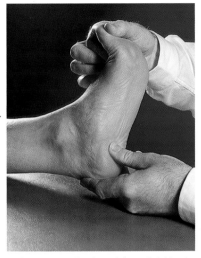

Fig. 6.1 Examination of the painful heel

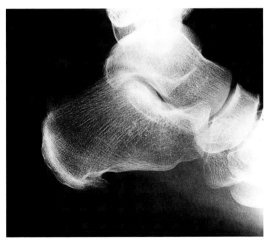

Fig. 6.2 Lateral radiograph of left heel

Plantar heel pain syndrome

1. Plantar heel pain syndrome (also known as plantar fasciitis or heel spur syndrome) is a common condition occurring at any time of life. It is seen in runners but also in less active patients. The 40–60-year age group is most frequently affected and the condition is more prevalent in obese individuals.

2. Pain after sleep and rest may be explained by contraction of the relaxed plantar fascia, which is then suddenly stretched on weightbearing.

3. The exact site of tenderness is located by first applying tension to the plantar fascia. This is best done by dorsiflexion of the great toe (Hick's Windlass effect) and then running the thumb from distal to proximal along the medial aspect of its central portion (Fig. 6.1). Firm pressure is then applied with a thumb over the medial calcaneal tuberosity and the pain elicited is diagnostic of the condition.

4. The significance of plantar spurs is not clear (Fig. 6.2). They are common in the general population, increasing in frequency with age (they occur in 10–16% of those over 50 years). Heel spurs are likely to be part of a reparative process. They probably arise after minor tearing of the plantar fascia's attachment onto the heel which causes bleeding and heterotopic ossification. In general, heel spurs are considered a normal variant and an insignificant finding when they are small, well defined and with smooth, regular cortical contours.

5. Plantar heel pain syndrome is self-limiting but a number of therapies are advocated during the painful stages. Commercially available heel inserts are useful and may provide valuable shock absorption (Fig. 6.3). Valgus pads can be used, either alone or in combination with cushioning

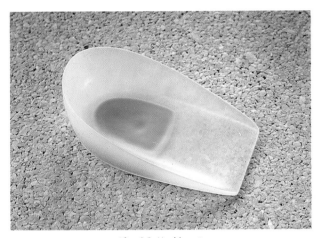

Fig. 6.3 Heel insert

and medial heel wedges or menisci (such as cobra pads), to limit foot pronation. Spread of the compressible heel pad can be contained by heel cups or an orthosis with a deep heel seat providing cushioning to the calcaneus. Stretching of the Achilles tendon by the use of nightsplints and exercises has also been advocated. Non-steroidal anti-inflammatory drugs and injection of corticosteroid may also help. Surgery to divide the plantar fascia (Steindler's release) is indicated only in extreme cases as it is detrimental to foot function.

Clinical tip

The authors locate the site of maximal tenderness, then insert the needle at an angle to the skin until bone is met. The needle is then withdrawn slightly, the syringe aspirated and the solution injected: methyl prednisolone 0.5 ml (40 mg) and lignocaine hydrochloride 0.5 ml 2% (Fig. 6.4).

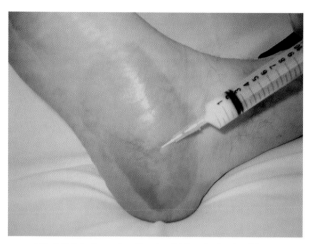

Fig. 6.4 Injection of corticosteroid for plantar fasciitis

KEY POINTS

- Plantar heel pain syndrome is typically seen as an overuse injury in runners, or in well built patients of middle age.

- Calcaneal spurs are common and are the result, rather than the cause, of plantar heel pain syndrome.

- Injections of corticosteroid appear to help in the short term.

- A variety of orthoses may be helpful during the painful phase of this self-limiting condition.

FURTHER READING

Crawford F, Atkins D, Young P, Edwards J (1999) Steroid injection for heel pain: evidence of short-term effectiveness. A randomized controlled trial. British Society for Rheumatology 38:974–7.

Crawford F, Atkins D, Edwards J (2000) Interventions for treating plantar heel pain (Cochrane review). In: The Cochrane Library, Issue 1, Oxford: Update software.

Daly PJ, Kitaoka HB, Chao EYS (1992) Plantar fasciotomy for intractable plantar fasciitis: clinical results and biomechanical evaluation. Foot and Ankle 13:188–95.

Probe RA, Baca BM, Adams R, Preece C (1999) Night splint treatment for plantar fasciitis: a prospective randomised study. Clinical Orthopaedics and Related Research 368: 190–5.

CASE 7

A 45-year-old lady presents with pain behind her heel after country dancing. Inspection reveals heel swelling (Fig. 7.1).

1. What are the differential diagnoses of these swellings and what predisposing factors are relevant? Which common synonyms are used to describe swellings at this site?

2. Will simply inserting a heel lift in the shoe help?

3. What operative interventions might be appropriate?

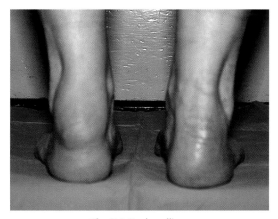

Fig. 7.1 Heel swelling

Achilles tendon bursitis

1. Three separate and different conditions may lead to swelling and pain at the heel. In this case the swelling is fusiform and lies in the line of the tendon itself. At surgery, the tendon was found to be chronically thickened and the sheath contained an excess of synovial fluid. The patient had rheumatoid arthritis. More commonly, the swelling overlies a bony prominence at the apex of the calcaneus (Fig. 7.2). Whether this is simply an anatomical variant of the bone or a consequence of recurrent traction on the calcaneal apophysis is unknown. The condition is termed Haglund's syndrome and in the US the prominence is commonly referred to as a 'pump bump'. The swelling may lie between the heel and tendon in which case it is termed a retrocalcaneal bursitis or may be primarily a superficial Achilles bursitis (Fig. 7.3).

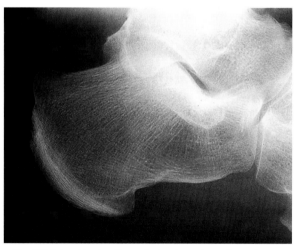

Fig. 7.2 Lateral heel radiograph showing calcaneal prominence

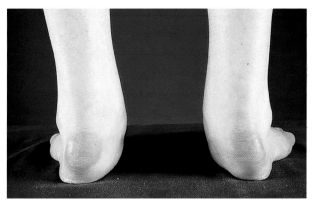

Fig. 7.3 Superficial Achilles bursitis

2. Heel elevation helps to relieve symptoms by tipping the calcaneus anteriorly, decreasing the pitch angle (the angle between the tangent to the plantar surface of the calcaneus and the horizontal). To an extent the foot will also slide forward in the shoe, taking pressure off the projection.

3. If symptoms persist despite heel elevation, then the prominence must be resected, or a wedge osteotomy constructed to turn it in towards the talus (Fig. 7.4a and b).

KEY POINTS

- Haglund's syndrome may include Achilles peritendinitis, retrocalcaneal bursitis and a 'pump' (Haglund's) bump.
- Aspiration and steroid injection may be useful in retrocalcaneal bursitis but are never performed for superficial bursitis. Patients *must* be made aware of the potential risk of subsequent tendon rupture.
- Resection of a heel bump is generally possible through a direct lateral approach.

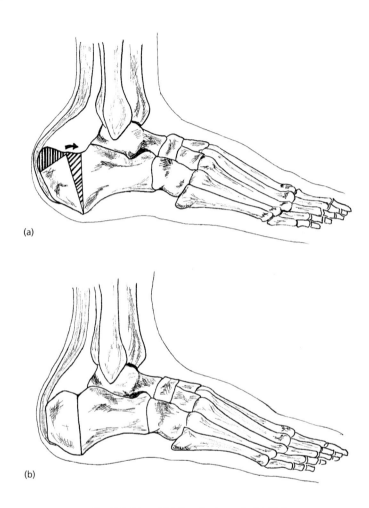

(a)

(b)

Fig. 7.4 (a) and (b) Dorsal calcaneal osteotomy

FURTHER READING

Heneghan MA, Pavlov H (1984) The Haglund painful heel syndrome: experimental investigation of cause and therapeutic implications. Clinical Orthopedics 187:228–34.

Keck SW, Kelly PJ (1965) Bursitis of the posterior part of the heel. Journal of Bone and Joint Surgery 47-A:1267–73.

CASE 8

The patient in Case 1 continues to complain of severe pain despite use of a hallux limitus plate. It is suggested that osteophyte trimming might be helpful (Fig. 8.1).

1. What is this operation called?

2. Are there any other alternative simple surgical procedures?

3. What is the optimal angle of joint arthrodesis? Are there any contraindications to fusion?

4. Is there a place for joint arthroplasty?

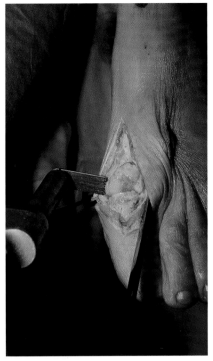

Fig. 8.1 Excision of dorsal osteophytes MTP joint

Surgery of hallux rigidus

1. Resection of the dorsal osteophytic lip is termed dorsal cheilectomy. Theoretically, the procedure allows the proximal phalanx to ride up over the metatarsal head in extension. In the authors' experience patients only gain short-term benefit from this operation.

2. In 1958, Kessel and Bonney reported the use of a dorsal flexion osteotomy at the base of the proximal phalanx to relieve the pain of hallux rigidus in adolescents. Patients were noted to retain plantar flexion of their toes, probably because of a developmental elevation of their first metatarsal, but to have lost dorsiflexion. Surgery transfers the arc of movement dorsally, improving toe function (Fig. 8.2). The condition is not common in adolescents and the operation is rarely performed.

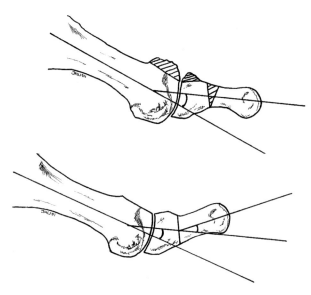

Fig. 8.2 Dorsal extension osteotomy

3. Arthrodesis remains the most popular surgical procedure for hallux rigidus. Ideally the toe should be fused with 10–15° dorsiflexion relative to the sole of the foot, equating to a bone MTP angle of 20–25°. A flexion angle at the top end of this range is required in women wishing to wear a high-heeled shoe. The relief of their pain undoubtedly pleases many patients, but consequently there is complete loss of joint mobility and a long-term tendency for patients to overload the lateral side of their feet. Arthritis of the IP joint is a contraindication to MTP fusion, as pain from the distal joint will become intolerable. Fusion of both joints is inadvisable as the patient will be left with neither proprioception nor toe-grip.

Several methods are commonly used to stabilize the arthrodesis until its union, but the authors have found that all of these will fail in some subjects, especially those with poor peripheral circulation. Indeed, the incidence of secondary surgery may be as high as 20% and patients should be forewarned. Of the methods available, holding the fusion by a circlage wire and a crossed Kirschner wire provides more rotational stability than insertion of a single cortical screw (Fig. 8.3a and b).

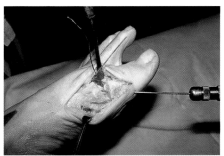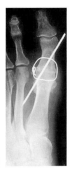

(a) (b)

Fig. 8.3 (a) and (b) MTP joint arthrodesis

4. The most common alternative to fusion of the first MTP joint remains a resection arthroplasty (Keller's procedure). Postoperative function will be acceptable in the elderly, but many younger patients find that their short toe is floppy and that they greatly miss the inherent stability afforded by a normal hallux.

In the past few years, there has been a trend towards joint replacement rather than fusion. There have been reports of fairly good long-term results using both hinged and phalangeal peg Silastic implants. Unfortunately, some patients develop severe granulomatous reactions to any Silastic debris, causing device loosening and ultimately failure (Fig. 8.4). Total joint arthroplasty, with a low friction metal on high density polyethylene bearing, is a more attractive proposition. Reasonable functional results are now being reported from the small number of implants on the market although, as with

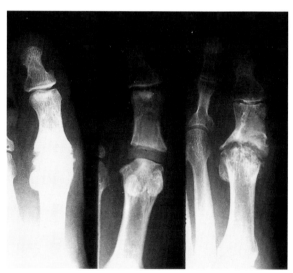

Fig. 8.4 Silastic hinge prosthesis at implantation and 15 years later

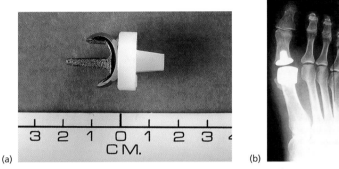

Fig. 8.5 (a) and (b) Total joint arthroplasty (Biomet®)

fusion, the authors have found that it may be at least 9 months after surgery before patients regain a normal gait (see Fig. 8.5).

KEY POINTS

- Fusion is the gold standard for treatment.
- IP arthritis is an absolute contraindication to MTP fusion.
- Total joint arthroplasty may be a valid alternative in the future.

FURTHER READING

Kessel L, Bonney G (1958) Hallux rigidus in the adolescent. Journal of Bone and Joint Surgery 40-B: 668–73.

O'Doherty DP, Lowrie IG, Magnussen PA et al. (1990) The management of the painful first metatarsophalangeal joint in the older patient: arthrodesis or Keller's arthroplasty? Journal of Bone and Joint Surgery 72-B:839–42.

Phillips JE, Hooper G (1986) A simple technique for arthrodesis of the first metatarsophalangeal joint. Journal of Bone and Joint Surgery 68-B:774–5.

Swanson AB (1972) Implant arthroplasty in disabilities of the great toe. In: Cacausland WR (ed.) American Academy of Orthopaedic Surgeons Instructional Course Lectures XXI. St Louis, MO, CV Mosby: 227–35.

Thomas PJ, Smith RW (1999) Proximal phalanx osteotomy for the surgical treatment of hallux rigidus. Foot and Ankle International 20:3–12.

CASE 9

Patients complaining of forefoot pain are often found to have callosities under their metatarsal heads. A 70-year-old man presents complaining that he feels he is 'walking on pebbles' (Fig. 9.1).

1. What factors might have contributed to the development of this condition?

2. Why did the callosities develop and what is the actual source of pain?

3. How might the surgeon endeavour to relieve the patient's symptoms if all conservative treatments have failed?

4. What long-term result may be expected from surgery?

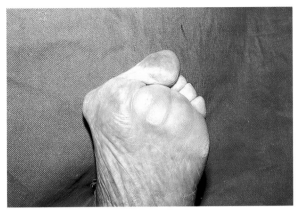

Fig. 9 .1 Forefoot callosities

Metatarsalgia

1. This patient initially presented to his general practitioner with hammering of his toes. The significance of MTP joint subluxation (Fig. 9.2) was not recognized and an insole was of no benefit and not worn. It was only a matter of time before pressure erosions developed. Indeed, it might be argued that the hammering of the digit only arose because of alteration of the normal weight distribution across the forefoot as ageing occurred and the metatarsal heads splayed. Similar progressive deformity would have developed had the patient suffered from rheumatoid arthritis.

2. Callosities develop as the subcutaneous tissues underlying the metatarsal heads atrophy. These changes are exacerbated by displacement of the plantar fat pad distally. Pain arises from the effects of direct pressure on the sole, metatarsal bursitis and joint synovitis.

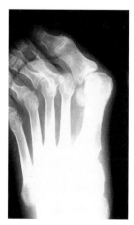

Fig. 9.2 Joint subluxation

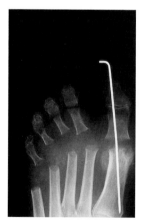

Fig. 9.3 Modified Fowler's procedure (Clayton)

3. The fundamental objective of any surgery is to produce a smooth 'arc' across the metatarsal bed. This may be achieved by selective shortening of the lesser metatarsals by an oblique Helal type osteotomy, allowing the metatarsal heads to slide dorsally. Usually, however, it is necessary to manufacture some form of procedure that will bring the plantar fat pad back into its rightful position. In this instance, the metatarsal condyles and proximal phalanges were resected through a dorsal approach (Fig. 9.3). It was felt that the vitality of the plantar skin was inadequate to allow resection of an ellipse of skin as originally described by Fowler. Kates' procedure (Fig. 9.4) would have had a lesser corrective effect on the toe hammering and Lipscomb's proximal phalangeal excision plus condylectomy (Fig. 9.5) would have left the second metatarsal long.

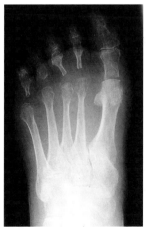

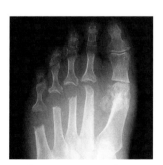

Fig. 9.4 Kates, Kessel, Kay procedure

Fig. 9.5 Lipscomb's procedure

4. The majority of patients are pleased with the early results of their surgery. They generally walk better and often are able to wear normal shoes for the first time in many years. Problems do arise, however, with time. In particular, patients may complain of progressive malalignment of the great toe, and the relative merits of hallux MTP fusion and Keller's resection have not been well defined. Some patients complain of recurrent callosities across the plantar arch and a radiograph may reveal that the end of the metatarsals have 'spiked'. A further local resection is often beneficial.

KEY POINTS

- Callosities form as the plantar fat pad is displaced distally.
- In rheumatoid arthritis the plantar skin will be atrophic.
- The surgeon must seek to provide a smooth metatarsal 'arc'.
- Partial phalangeal resection may be necessary if the toes are clawed.

FURTHER READING

Fowler AW (1959) A method of forefoot reconstruction. Journal of Bone and Joint Surgery 41-B:507–13.

Helal B (1975) Metatarsal osteotomy for metatarsalgia. Journal of Bone and Joint Surgery 57-B:187–92.

Karbowski A, Schwitalle M, Eckhardt A (1998) Arthroplasty of the forefoot in rheumatoid arthritis: long-term results after Clayton procedure. Acta Orthopaedic Belgica 64:401–5.

Kates A, Kessel L, Kay A (1967) Arthroplasty of the forefoot. Journal of Bone and Joint Surgery 49-B:552–7.

Lipscomb RR, Benson GM, Sones DA (1972) Resection of proximal phalanges and metatarsal condyles for deformities of the forefoot due to rheumatoid arthritis. Clinical Orthopedics 82:24–31.

CASE 10

A 58-year-old man presents with a swelling on his great toe 'the size of a golf ball' (Fig. 10.1). Normally, when it reached that size he stated that his toe would become uncomfortable and he would resort to piercing the swelling with a pin, expressing a gelatinous fluid like 'egg white'. He wondered whether he might find a more permanent cure.

1. What is the 'egg white' fluid that is expressed from the swelling and therefore what is the diagnosis?

2. What is the aetiopathology of this condition?

3. What should be done for this patient?

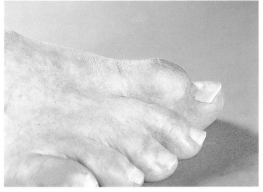

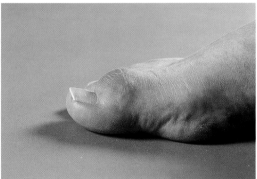

Fig. 10.1 Swelling on right hallux

Ganglion

1. The description of the fluid is characteristic of synovial fluid, suggesting a ganglion cyst. A ganglion presents as a swelling that is soft and fluctuant to the touch.

2. Ganglion cysts are fluid-filled sacs arising through herniation of a joint capsule or synovial sheath. They are commonly found on the dorsum of the foot because of the number of synovial sheaths passing around the ankle (Fig. 10.2). They also occur as pea-like swellings in the flexor tendon sheaths of the toes. When illuminated, these fluid-filled tumours will disperse light in contrast to opaque solid masses, which should be viewed with suspicion.

3. If asymptomatic and small then ganglia are best left alone. Ganglia that become large or uncomfortable, as in the case illustrated above, should be aspirated to provide the patient with at least temporary relief of the symptoms. The patient should, however, be informed that the rate of recurrence from aspiration alone will be in excess of 70%. This may be reduced

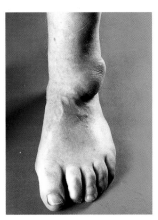

Fig. 10.2 Ganglion over dorsolateral ankle joint

by corticosteroid injection. Excision of the lesion (Fig. 10.3) will provide a more certain result, provided that care is taken to ensure that the entire cyst wall is removed, but even then recurrences can occur and patients should be warned accordingly.

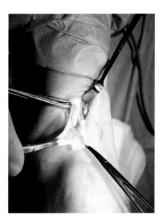

Fig. 10.3 Surgical excision of a dorsal ankle ganglion

KEY POINTS

- Ganglia are common occurrences on the dorsum of the foot.
- Ganglia are benign lesions arising through herniation of a joint capsule or tendon sheath.
- Asymptomatic lesions do not require intervention.
- Large and uncomfortable swellings can be aspirated, but excision will often be required.

FURTHER READING

Slavitt JA, Behesht F, Lenet M, Sherman M (1980) Ganglions of the foot: a six year retrospective study and a review of the literature. Journal of the American Podiatric Medicine Association 70:459–65.

CASE 11

Patients generally present to the clinic with lesser deformity than that shown in Case 5. The radiograph below was taken of a 46-year-old secretary's foot (Fig. 11.1). She was simply troubled when she wore tight-fitting shoes, but had no pain at other times.

1. If the hallux valgus were to be addressed, what type of realignment should be performed?

2. Is there any place for a Keller's resection arthroplasty?

3. Can the displacement of the sesamoids shown be discounted?

4. Following surgery, when could the lady reasonably expect to be symptom free?

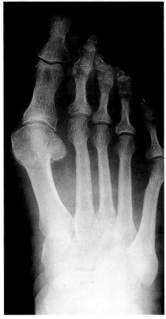

Fig. 11.1 Moderate hallux valgus

Surgery of hallux valgus

1. The authors believe that it is essential to maintain 'joint height' when performing a metatarsal osteotomy. Thus, if the first metatarsal is already short then any further shortening is ill advised. In the vast majority of individuals the intermetatarsal angle will be less than 15° and the deformity may be corrected by a distal osteotomy preserving length (Fig. 11.2a and b). Excessive metatarsus primus varus will require some form of shaft realignment as part of, or in addition to, metatarsal head displacement (Fig. 11.3).

2. The hallux is shortened and left 'floppy' after Keller's resection arthroplasty (removal of the proximal third of the

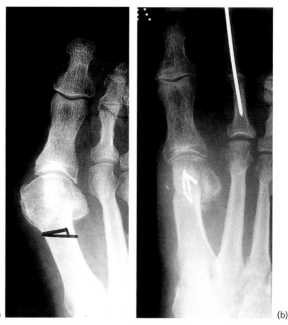

(a)

(b)

Fig. 11.2 (a) and (b) Mitchell's osteotomy

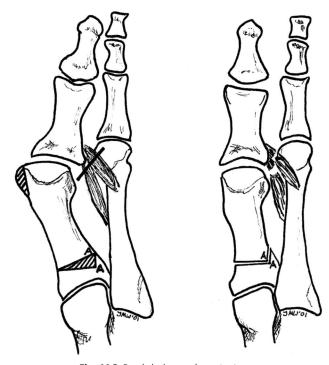

Fig. 11.3 Basal closing wedge osteotomy

proximal phalanx). It is not uncommon for the toe to 'cock-up' (Fig. 11.4) and the loss of digit stability often leads to metatarsalgia because of disruption of the attachments of the plantar fascia and intrinsic muscles. The majority of young patients will not accept the inherent loss of 'push-off'. The authors would therefore only consider this procedure for inactive patients in late middle age, presenting with significant MTP joint arthritis.

3. The sesamoids, bound into flexor hallucis brevis, tend to retain their position as the hallux deviates medially. Since the central ridge on the underside of the metatarsal head may

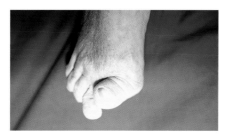

Fig. 11.4 Toe after Keller's resection arthroplasty

have flattened off as the medial sesamoid translocates, simply realigning the metatarsal may not be sufficient to restore the sesamoid to its natural position. A reefing of the medial joint capsule and sesamoidal ligament is usually required.

4. Most patients will be pleased with the results of corrective surgery provided that first metatarsal length is preserved. Union of any osteotomy will take a minimum of 6 weeks and often takes up to 12. We recommend immobilization of the foot in a fibreglass sabot cast for 6 weeks even if fixation is secure (Fig. 11.5). Malunion of the osteotomy is then less

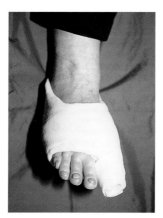

Fig. 11.5 Fibreglass sabot cast

likely and we find that patients are more comfortable and in consequence generally more mobile.

KEY POINTS

- Shortening of the first metatarsal should be avoided.
- An attempt should be made to restore the sesamoids to their position below the metatarsal head.
- Long-term results of surgery are generally good.

FURTHER READING

Ferrari J, Higgins JP, Williams RL (2001) Interventions for treating hallux valgus (abductovalgus) and bunions (Cochrane review). In: The Cochrane Library, Issue 1, Oxford: Update software.

Fokter SK, Podobnik J, Vengust V (1999) Late results of modified Mitchell procedure for the treatment of hallux valgus. Foot and Ankle International 20:296–300.

Judge MS, LaPointe S, Yu GV, Shook JE, Taylor RP (1999) The effect of hallux abducto-valgus surgery on the sesamoid apparatus position. Journal of the American Podiatric Medicine Association 89:551–9.

Trnka HJ, Zembsch A, Easley ME, Salzer M, Ritschl P, Myerson MS (2000) The chevron osteotomy for correction of hallux valgus. Comparison of findings after two and five years of follow-up. Journal of Bone and Joint Surgery 82-A:1373–8.

Zembsch A, Trnka HJ, Ritschl P (2000) Correction of hallux valgus. Metatarsal osteotomy versus excision arthroplasty. Clinical Orthopedics 376:183–94.

CASE 12

For 6 months a 45-year-old bank manager complained that he had experienced pain under the inner arch of his foot when playing golf. Inspection revealed a lesion, shown in Figure 12.1.

1. This lump is painful. What would be a reasonable differential diagnosis?

2. There are certain factors predisposing to lesions of this type; can you name them?

3. Assuming that the lump was excised, what might be the end result?

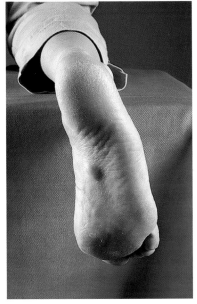

Fig. 12.1 Lesion in the sole of left foot

ORTHOPAEDICS

Plantar fibroma

1. The lesion shown is typical of a nodule arising within the plantar fascia (Fig. 12.2). There are actually very few other conditions which might produce a similarly tender nodule. Granulomas may occur around a foreign body, but the patient is usually aware of preceding trauma. The only other lesion of note, assuming that there is no underlying bony abnormality, is a neurilemmoma (Schwannoma: tumour of a peripheral nerve sheath) as shown in Figure 12.3.

2. Plantar fibromatosis is analogous to palmar fibromatosis (Dupuytren's disease) and it is generally accepted that they are one and the same condition. Histological analysis in the early stages will identify arrays of myofibroblasts, producing a lesion that tends to be fairly soft and may be exquisitely tender. At this stage, care has to be taken to ensure that the lesion is not mistaken for a fibrosarcoma. With maturity, these characteristics change as the nodule becomes much firmer because of a decrease in cell density and a laying down of collagen.

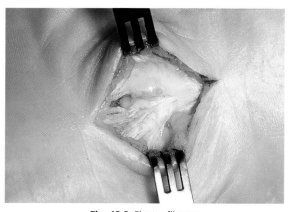

Fig. 12.2 Plantar fibroma

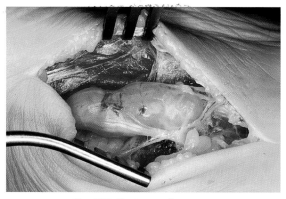

Fig. 12.3 Plantar neurilemmoma

The commonest identifiable factor predisposing to a plantar lesion is probably trauma. This may simply have been a tearing of the fibres of the ligament, similar to that causing plantar fasciitis, or a direct laceration. The fact that direct trauma will not always cause fibroma formation indicates that the patient must also have a predisposition to the condition. A genetic link is fairly well established, certainly in patients with a Dupuytren's palmar contracture. Affected subjects will often have a familial tendency to the condition and there is also an association with idiopathic epilepsy and excessive alcohol intake.

3. A conservative approach to treatment is generally recommended. With the passage of time the lesions become less acutely tender, although they never alter much in size. Steroid infiltration may reduce perinodular inflammation, but will not shrink the lesion *per se*. If a lesion becomes large then surgical excision may be requested. The patient should be warned that recurrence is likely, especially if the nodules are multiple, bilateral, or occur in patients with a strong family history. Since the lesion usually infiltrates the dermis a skin graft may be required.

KEY POINTS

- Plantar fibromatosis is common in Caucasians.
- The lesion consists of myofibroblasts linked to extracellular filaments.
- Treatment should be conservative if possible.
- Recurrence is frequent after surgical resection.

FURTHER READING

De Palma L, Santucci A, Gigante A, Di Giulio A, Carloni S (1999) Plantar fibromatosis: an immunohistochemical and ultrastructural study. Foot and Ankle International 20:253–7.

Sammarco GJ, Mangone PG (2000) Classification and treatment of plantar fibromatosis. Foot and Ankle International 21:563–9.

Dermatology

CASE 13

This 65-year-old lady has discoloration of the skin over her lower leg and medial ankle. She has been troubled by a recurrent ulcer in this area.

1. What is the underlying pathology shown in Figures 13.1 and 13.2?

2. Discuss the cause.

3. How is this managed?

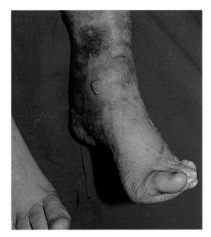

Fig. 13.1 Skin appearance

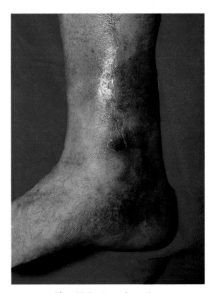

Fig. 13.2 Leg ulceration

Venous ulceration

1. Varicose eczema/ulceration (gravitational eczema) presents in elderly patients with venous hypertension. The venous insufficiency results in a rise in capillary hydrostatic pressure and permeability, interfering with the diffusion of nutrients and resulting in tissue necrosis. Fibrin is deposited as a pericapillary cuff around the ankle. This is termed lipodermatosclerosis.

2. Brown haemosiderin deposits from extravasated red cells, telangiectasia and white lacy scars (atrophie blanche) occur over the medial malleolus. Minor trauma to eczematous skin often leads to ulceration (Fig. 13.2).

3. Treatment of venous ulcers is aimed at reducing venous hypertension with the use of elevation and compression bandages. Walking should be encouraged (and standing discouraged) to improve the muscle pump. Ulcer healing is a slow protracted process, which can be aided with a variety of wound dressings. Oral therapy includes the use of diuretics, antibiotics and stanozolol.

KEY POINTS

- Venous insufficiency is characterized by discoloration and varicose eczema on the lower leg.
- Ulcers follow minor trauma.
- Venous ulcer healing is protracted.

FURTHER READING

Moffat C, O'Hare L (1995) Graduated compression hosiery for venous ulceration. Journal of Wound Care 4(10):41–59.

CASE 14

A middle-aged woman presents with a persistent, red scaly rash on the outer aspect of her foot (Fig. 14.1). As can be seen in the figure, there are yellow pustules present. She has similar lesions on the palms of her hands, both of which have been present for a considerable time. She is a smoker.

Younger patients often also present with erythematous lesions. The lesion shown in Figure 14.2 occurred in a young boy who was keen on sport and always wore training shoes.

1. Give the diagnosis for the first condition.

2. What is responsible for the erythematous lesion in the second condition?

3. What treatment would be appropriate in both instances?

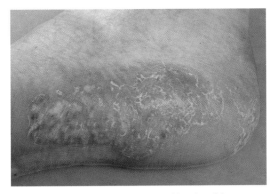

Fig. 14.1 Skin lesion on lateral border of foot

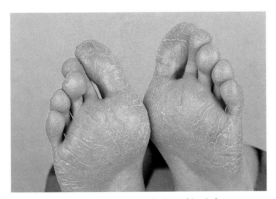

Fig. 14.2 Erythematous lesion of both feet

Plantar pustulosis/dermatosis

1. Palmoplantar pustulosis is a localized form of psoriasis which is confined to the palms and soles of middle-aged patients who invariably smoke. It frequently occurs without evidence of psoriasis elsewhere. It is characterized by sterile yellowish-white pustules that desiccate to leave discrete yellow-to-brown coloured stains. The surrounding skin is inflamed and scaly. Typically plantar pustulosis is seen along the medial longitudinal arches of the feet.

2. Juvenile plantar dermatosis is a scaly, glazed, fissured erythema seen on the weightbearing areas of the feet, mainly across the forefoot. The skin is drier than in adult pustulosis and the condition is considered to be a contact dermatitis to synthetic materials.

3. Plantar pustulosis follows a protracted course and is often resistant to treatments such as coal tar, dithranol and steroids, although potent steroids and ultraviolet radiation may be beneficial. Treatment of the juvenile condition is easier, as often the children will be found wearing socks and shoes made from synthetic materials. They should try using an emollient cream such as Unguentum Merck and wear leather shoes if possible.

KEY POINTS

- Plantar pustulosis is a form of psoriasis seen on the feet.
- Juvenile plantar dermatosis is a contact dermatitis caused by synthetic footwear.
- Erythematous lesions are managed with steroids and emollients.

FURTHER READING

Graham R (1989) Palmo-plantar pustulosis. Practitioner 233:1428–39.

Yiannias JA, Winkelmann RK, Connolly SM (1998) Contact sensitivities in palmar plantar pustulosis. Contact Dermatitis 39:108–11.

CASE 15

This male patient worked in the mines for many years. He is now 74 years old and regularly attends for podiatric care of his nails. On examination, all his nails are thickened and discoloured (Fig. 15.1). He also has macerated skin between his fourth and fifth toes and there is a red scaly patch on the side of his right foot (Fig. 15.2).

1. Why is the condition of this ex-miner's toenails related to his previous work?

2. In more equivocal cases how should diagnosis be confirmed?

3. Is the condition of the nails associated with the scaly patch on the right foot (Fig. 15.2)?

4. Do the nails and skin condition require treatment and if so, with what?

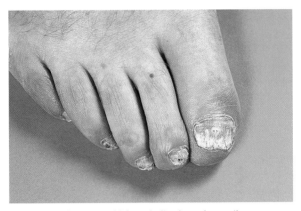

Fig. 15.1 Thickened, discoloured toenails

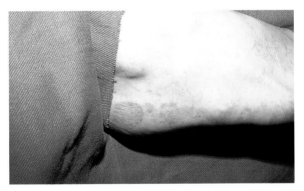

Fig. 15.2 Scaly patch on lateral border of right foot

Fungal foot infections

1. This man has a fungal infection of his nails (onychomycosis, tinea unguium). Fungal nails are an occupational hazard of miners because they share communal bathing facilities. Fungal nail infections are caused by dermatophytes which digest keratin by producing enzymes. There are three genera of dermatophytes: *Microsporum*, *Trichophyton* and *Epidermophyton*. *Trichophyton rubrum* is the most common species of dermatophyte to infect the nails. The nail plate becomes thickened, separated from the nail bed, discoloured, brittle and develops a honeycombed structure. The fungus affects one or more nails, but rarely all of them; this man being the exception to the rule. The condition is more common with increasing age.

2. In more equivocal cases, diagnosis can be confirmed by the finding of hyphae on microscopy. To identify a specific dermatophyte the fungus must be cultured.

3. The scaly patch is athlete's foot (ringworm, tinea pedis), which is also caused by a superficial fungal infection similar to that seen in Figure 15.1.

4. Only occasionally do fungal nails require treatment. This man was not troubled with his toenails and did not require treatment other than reassurance and palliative nail care. However, younger patients, especially women, can be more self-conscious of discoloured thickened toenails and are more likely to request treatment. Treatment of fungal nails requires systemic medication although amorolfine (Loceryl) is a nail lacquer that has some effect. Terbinafine (Lamisil) is an oral fungicidal which is now the mainstay of therapy for fungal nails, superseding griseofulvin. Treatment should be continued for a full 3 months to eradicate the infection.

Skin infection is more likely to respond to topical antifungal applications. In the first instance, patients should be given advice to dry their feet well after bathing, particularly between their toes. The use of astringents will reduce the moisture content of the skin and therefore the risk of infection. A topical agent such as Whitfield's ointment, although old-fashioned, is still useful but has been largely superseded by drugs of the azole (clotrimazole Canesten, miconazole Daktarin) and allylamine (terbinafine Lamisil) groups. Recent research suggests that there is little difference in efficacy between azoles and allylamines, although the latter are more expensive.

KEY POINTS

- Fungal infections of the skin and nails are common, affecting about 10% of the population.
- They are caused by dermatophyte infections.
- Skin and nail infections are often found together.
- Infection of the skin requires advice and astringents or, if persistent, azoles or allylamines.

FURTHER READING

Gentles JC, Evans EGV (1973) Foot infections in swimming baths. British Medical Journal 3(5874):260–2.

Hart R, Bell-Syer SE, Crawford F, Torgerson D, Young P, Russell IT (1999) Systematic review of topical treatments for fungal infections of the skin and nails of the feet. British Medical Journal 319:79–82.

CASE 16

A young student is troubled with a painful ingrowing toenail. Her trouble first began when she cut down the side of her nail. As can be seen in Figure 16.1, her toe is infected and there is hypergranulation tissue present. She has had three courses of Flucloxacillin. Each course brought about resolution of her infection but only for a few weeks.

1. Two distinct types of ingrowing toenail are recognized. Can you name them and what type does this young woman have?

2. Why do the antibiotics only have a short-term effect?

3. Surgically, how is this painful nail condition best treated?

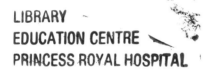

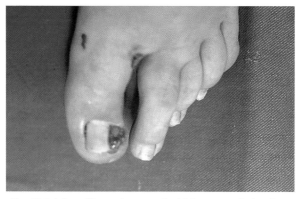

Fig. 16.1 Infected ingrowing toenail with hypergranulation tissue

Ingrowing toenails

1. Ingrowing toenails are a painful condition in which the nail edge penetrates the nail fold. There are two main causes. Ingrowth may be caused by a splinter of nail penetrating the nail sulcus (onychocryptosis), as presented on the previous page. This is more likely to occur if the nail plate is thin and broad, and is often accompanied by secondary infection and hypergranulation tissue. This type of nail problem is seen more often in young adult men and may be precipitated by poor nail cutting. Figure 16.2 shows an onychocryptosis with the spike of nail growing distally out of the end of the toe.

In older women, where footwear may be a contributory factor, ingrowing toenails are caused by an increased transverse curvature of the nail (involuted or incurvature of the nail: Fig. 16.3). They are less likely to become infected but painful keratosis may develop in the nail folds. Poor management of these inwardly curved nails can lead to a spike of the involuted nail penetrating the skin as in onychocryptosis above.

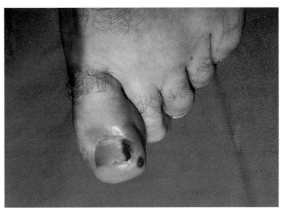

Fig. 16.2 Severe onychocryptosis with spike penetrating the end of the toe

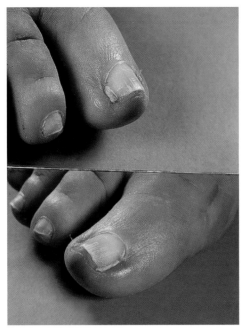

Fig. 16.3 Involution (incurvature) of the nail

2. Treatment of onychocryptosis with antibiotics resolves the immediate problem of infection but only temporarily, as the complaint soon recurs unless the offending portion of nail is removed. Removal of the nail splinter and simultaneous narrowing will bring about a more satisfactory outcome. Removal of the entire nail is considered when the curvature of the toenail is too great or excessively thick (onychauxis or onychogryposis) and if fungal infection of the nail plate is present (onychomycosis).

3. Evidence shows that removal of part or the entire nail with phenolization is better than surgical excision alone (Zadik's or Winograd's procedures). Both Zadik's and Winograd's (wedge excision) necessitate a more extensive approach and wound suture, and are generally more painful for the patient postoperatively; there is a high risk of regrowth of spikes of nail and thus failure of the procedure (Fig. 16.4).

The main benefit of phenol application is the reduced need for further operation because of recurrent nail growth; however, there is also less postoperative pain and bleeding. Furthermore, simple removal of the nail with phenolization is not precluded by the presence of infection and does not require sutures. On the downside, it should be remembered that phenol is caustic and should be handled with extreme care. Phenol is also damaging to the wound tissues and may give rise to prolonged wound healing, increasing the risk of postoperative infection. These disadvantages are greatly outweighed by the advantages listed above.

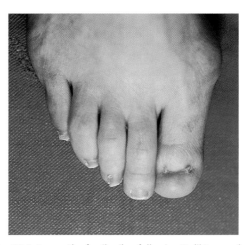

Fig. 16.4 Regrowth of nail spikes following Zadik's procedure

Clinical tip: partial removal of the toenail with phenolization for onychocryptosis

Apply an exsanguinating tourniquet (Esmarch bandage) around the toe. Identify the portion of nail to be removed. Separate this portion of nail plate from the nail bed and split the nail with a sharp chisel blade (Fig. 16.5a and b). Use forceps to gain a firm hold on the portion of nail and gently rotate towards the centre of the toe. Ensure that the nail matrix has been removed intact. Then, having applied Vaseline along the skin margin to protect it, apply 80% strength phenol to the germinal matrix with a fine cotton bud and rub in well (Fig. 16.5c). Apply for a minimum of 3 minutes, then irrigate the nail fold with alcohol or saline solution. Dress the toe firstly with paraffin tulle gauze, then gauze swabs and secure with a tubular bandage. Figure 16.6 shows the result 4 weeks after operation.

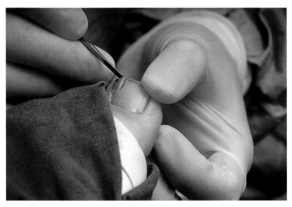

(a)

Fig. 16.5 (a)–(b) Removal of a lateral section of toenail. (c) Phenolization of germinal matrix

Fig. 16.5 (b) and (c), see overleaf

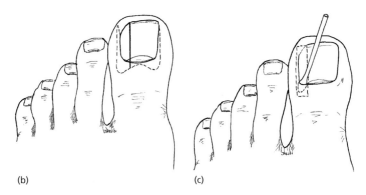

(b)   (c)

Fig. 16.5 (*continued*)

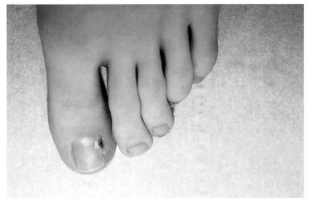

Fig. 16.6 Same toe as shown in Fig. 16.1, 4 weeks after partial removal and phenolization

KEY POINTS

- Ingrowing toenails differ in aetiology in young and old patients.
- Antibiotics will only bring about short-term relief if the nail margin is not removed.
- Phenolization of the nail matrix is recommended after removal of the toenail.

FURTHER READING

Laxton C (1995) Clinical audit of forefoot surgery performed by registered medical practitioners and podiatrists. Journal of Public Health Medicine 17:311–17.

Rounding C, Hulm S (1999) Surgical treatments for ingrowing toenails (Cochrane review). In: The Cochrane Library, Issue 4. Oxford: Update software.

Van Der Ham AC, Hackeng CAH, Yo TI (1990) The treatment of ingrowing toenails: a randomised comparison of wedge excision and phenol cauterisation. Journal of Bone and Joint Surgery 72-B:507–9.

CASE 17

A teenage girl presents with a painful big toenail. The pain is exacerbated with certain footwear and with direct pressure on the nail plate. The nail plate has separated from the nail bed and the lesion has been discharging (Fig. 17.1a and b). As a result, she has received two courses of antibiotics. This girl's mother is convinced that this is an ingrowing toenail and she has sought podiatry treatment for her.

1. Why is this girl's mother wrong in her assessment of this nail problem and what are your differential diagnoses?

2. What is the cause of this nail condition?

3. How would you confirm your diagnosis?

4. What is the correct management of this condition?

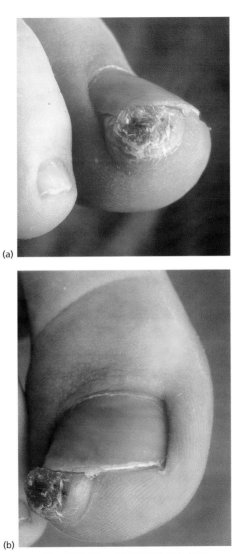

(a)

(b)

Fig. 17.1 (a) and (b) Raised nail plate

Subungual exostosis

1. A firm swelling appears under the nail plate, raising it from the nail bed. Compare this with the ingrowing toenail in Figure 16.1 where hypergranulation tissue forms at the nail folds. This therefore is a subungual exostosis. Other differential diagnoses would be a subungual wart, corn, malignant melanoma or periungual fibroma (Fig. 17.2).

2. Subungual exostosis is a benign tumour of trabecular bone with a fibrocartilage cap. It presents most frequently in teenagers and young adults. Exostoses are reputed to be caused by trauma, but there is no strong evidence for this and most patients do not report a traumatic incidence. In 70% of cases the great toe is affected.

3. Diagnosis is confirmed by X-ray. Histology demonstrates a stalk of normal trabecular bone capped with fibrocartilage (Fig. 17.3).

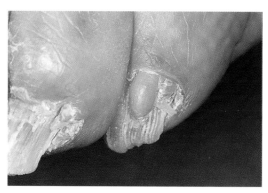

Fig. 17.2 Periungual fibroma of proximal nail fold

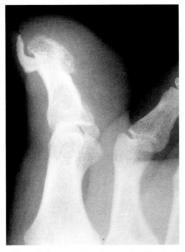

Fig. 17.3 Lateral radiograph of hallux

4. Complete surgical excision is the treatment of choice. This can be performed on a day-care basis using a ring block anaesthetic (Fig. 17.4) and Esmarch tourniquet around the toe. The toenail is completely removed, preferably without

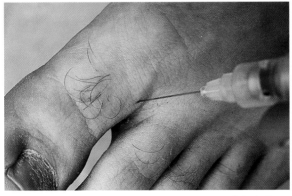

Fig. 17.4 Technique of local anaesthetic injection of the hallux

disturbing the nail matrix. The stalk of the exostosis is removed with bone rongeurs or a small osteotome, so that bone is removed from below the level of the normal periosteum. Sufficient bone must be removed to avoid recurrence (reported to be as high as 15% within 1 year). The wound should be left open and allowed to close by secondary intention.

Clinical tip: technique of hallux injection (ring block)

Use plain solutions of lignocaine hydrochloride (2%) 2–4 ml, or bupivacaine hydrochloride (0.5%) 1–2 ml. A dental needle (Fig. 17.4) is ideal but, failing this, a small diameter (blue) needle should be used. Identify the MTP and the IP joints and find the midpoint of the proximal phalanx. Always inject the lateral side of the toe first (Fig. 17.4), as this is less painful. Introduce the needle at an angle of 60° to the skin and insert the needle to the plantar side of the toe. Inject 0.5–1 ml of anaesthetic plantarward and the same dorsally. Repeat on the medial side.

KEY POINTS

- The great toenail is affected in 70% of cases.
- Pain arises where the nail plate becomes raised and distorted.
- X-rays confirm the diagnosis.
- Surgical excision is the treatment of choice.

FURTHER READING

David D, Cohen P (1996) Subungual exostosis: case report and review of the literature. Paediatric Dermatology 13:212–18.

De Berker D, Langtry J (1999) Treatment of subungual exostoses by elective day case surgery. British Journal of Dermatology 140:915–18.

CASE 18

This is a common skin lesion that has appeared suddenly on the sole of this young swimmer's foot (Fig. 18.1). It has been present for about 6 weeks and appears to be getting larger. The boy's mother is demanding treatment.

1. Name this skin lesion.

2. Briefly describe the pathology of this lesion.

3. Which group of patients is at greater risk of this skin condition?

4. Should this mother's demands be met and, if so, what treatment is advocated?

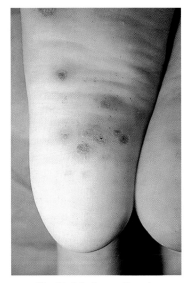

Fig. 18.1 Lesion on the sole

Viral warts

1. Plantar warts (verrucae) are common benign cutaneous tumours caused by infection of epidermal cells with human papilloma virus (HPV). Over 60 subtypes of DNA have been identified and HPV I, II and III are associated with plantar warts. They are seen in children and adolescents on the soles of the feet, where pressure causes them to grow into the dermis. Verrucae are more common in swimmers. The non-slip pool surfaces may macerate the skin, aiding inoculation of any free virus material. On the soles of the feet they can be difficult to distinguish from keratoses (corns) (Table 18.1).

2. The prickle cell layer of the epidermis becomes thickened and hyperkeratotic. Keratinocytes in the granular layer are vacuolated from infection with the wart virus.

3. Immunosuppressed individuals such as those with organ transplants are susceptible to viral warts. Mosaic warts are plaques on the soles that comprise multiple individual warts. These are indicative of poor natural resistance to infection and present a difficult challenge.

Table 18.1 Differentiation between a wart and a keratosis

Observation	Wart	Keratosis
After removal of overlying callus	Punctate spots (thrombosed capillaries), bleeding points	Skin concavity
Skin striae	Diverge from the lesion	Do not diverge
Site	Any site	Always weight-bearing site
Effect of lateral compression (pinching)	Very painful	Not painful

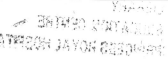

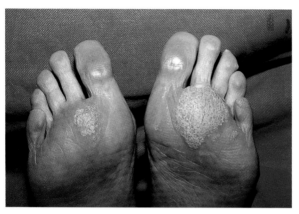

Fig. 18.2 Large mosaic warts on the soles of the feet in a patient undergoing cyclosporin therapy 5 years after a heart transplant

4. The decision as to whether to treat a verruca depends on the nature of the lesion. If it is painful, spreading, or growing larger, treatment is indicated. As this boy's lesion appears to be getting larger, then treatment with 20% salicylic acid (a keratolytic), or cryotherapy with either nitrous oxide or liquid nitrogen is indicated (Fig. 18.3). This may have to be repeated at fortnightly intervals on three or four occasions.

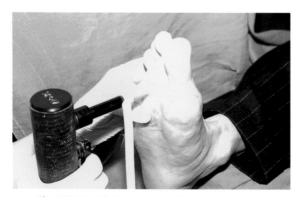

Fig. 18.3 Liquid nitrogen application to plantar warts

95

Warts generally resolve spontaneously within 6 months in children. However, in adults they can persist for longer and sometimes for many years. There is a school of thought that suggests that, in children, there is a value in allowing the body's immune system to be sensitized to the virus and therefore confer future immunity. As a rule of thumb, if plantar warts are painful, spreading, increasing in size or interfering with usual activities, then treatment is probably indicated. As this boy's lesion appears to be getting larger, then treatment should be considered.

There are a number of treatment options, none of which guarantee any form of success. The use of caustics and keratolytics have to be repeated at weekly intervals on several occasions and necessitate keeping the foot dry. A more painful, but potentially more convenient alternative, cryotherapy with either nitrous oxide or liquid nitrogen, aims to destroy the wart tissue by freezing. Homeopathic remedies such as Thuja and Kalanchoe are less harmful options which the patient can happily administer themselves but claims as to their efficacy remain anecdotal at this time.

Occasionally, antiviral therapy such as intralesional bleomycin or immunotherapy such as dinitrochlorobenzene (DNCB) or diphencyprone may be indicated for recalcitrant lesions in adults.

KEY POINTS

- Warts are common on the soles of the feet, particularly in children.
- Treatments include keratolytics and cryotherapy.
- Surface occlusion (e.g. verruca socks) will prevent 'contact' spread.

FURTHER READING

Bunney M (1983) Viral warts. Churchill Livingstone, Edinburgh.

Gibbs S, Harvey I, Sterling JC, Stark R (2001) Local treatments for cutaneous warts (Cochrane Review). In: The Cochrane Library, Issue 2, 2001 Oxford: Update software.

CASE 19

A 20-year-old male student presents with a long-standing problem affecting both his feet (Fig. 19.1). His GP had never seen this problem before and so referred the student to a dermatology clinic.

1. Give the diagnosis.

2. Which organism is responsible?

3. What is the treatment?

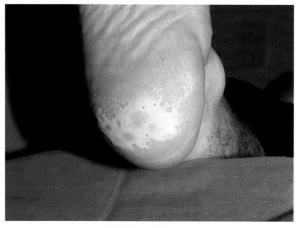

Fig. 19.1 Skin lesion on heel

Pitted keratolysis

1. Pitted keratolysis is a micrococcal infection caused by overgrowth of diphtheroid commensals. Keratin is resorbed, producing pitting of the skin.

2. Micrococci proliferate in moist conditions and patients with this complaint often sweat profusely (hyperhidrosis) and may wear occlusive footwear. There is usually an accompanying malodour.

3. The key to treatment is to deal with the hyperhidrosis. This student was treated successfully with formalin soaks. Other possible treatments include painting the skin with potassium permanganate or applying neomycin powder topically.

KEY POINTS

- Hyperhidrosis allows proliferation of skin pathogens.
- Pitted keratolysis is caused by a micrococcal infection.
- Hyperhidrosis is treated with astringents such as formalin or potassium permanganate soaks.

FURTHER READING

Takama H, Tamada Y, Yano K, Nitta Y, Ikeya T (1997) Pitted keratolysis: clinical manifestations in 53 cases. British Journal of Dermatology 137:282–5.

CASE 20

A middle-aged woman presents with chilblains and a history of painful, white fingers and toes on exposure to cold (Fig. 20.1).

1. What exactly is this condition?

2. With which connective tissue disorder is this condition associated?

3. How is the condition managed?

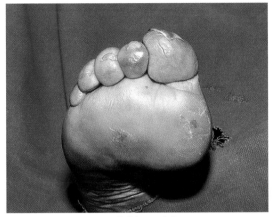

Fig. 20.1 Chilblains of the toes

Chilblains

1. Chilblains (perniosis) are a localized exaggerated response to cold, mostly affecting women and children, and commonly occurring on the fingers and toes. After exposure to cold there is prolonged constriction of the cutaneous arterioles and venules. The toes initially become red, hot and swollen because of a hyperaemic reaction and this is accompanied by intense itching. There follows a period of cyanosis and, if the circulation does not improve, then ulcers form.

2. Chilblains are most commonly evident in patients with Raynaud's phenomenon. This condition is characterized by paroxysmal vasoconstriction of the digital vessels, causing the fingers and toes to turn white (due to ischaemia), become cyanotic (due to capillary dilatation with a stagnant blood flow) and then turn red (due to reactive hyperaemia). When Raynaud's is idiopathic it is termed a disease and, when seen secondary to other conditions, it is termed a phenomenon. The disease is common. Ninety per cent of patients are women and there is often a family history. Raynaud's phenomenon is associated with other connective tissue diseases, notably in systemic sclerosis where a limited scleroderma may be associated with calcinosis, oesophageal involvement and telangiectasia – the CREST syndrome (see Fig. 20.2).

Other causes of Raynaud's are:

- Arterial occlusive conditions occurring in patients with atherosclerosis and Buerger's disease.
- Impaired vascular innervation occurring secondary to syringomyelia or paraplegia.
- Reflex vasoconstriction from occupational trauma, for example after prolonged typing or use of pneumatic tools.
- Bacterial toxins causing vasoconstriction.
- Increased blood viscosity.

002

2020

2000

0000

0000

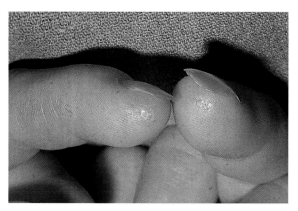

Fig. 20.2 Calcinosis cutis

3. Avoidance of cold is essential. Topical applications of 4% balsam of Peru are helpful but in many instances, where ulceration is recurrent, vasodilators such as the calcium channel blocker nifedipine may be required. Raynaud's is provoked by cold and therefore patients should be advised to keep their feet warm and avoid damp, cold conditions. In severe cases digital necrosis necessitates amputation.

KEY POINTS

- Chilblains are an exaggerated response to cold and are seen secondary to Raynaud's.
- Raynaud's is a vasoconstrictive disorder mainly affecting middle-aged women. It is associated with scleroderma in CREST syndrome.
- Avoidance of cold is essential and vasodilators may be required.

FURTHER READING

Dowd PM (1986) Nifedipine in the treatment of chilblains. British Medical Journal 293:923–40.

Kanwar AJ, Ghosh S, Dhar S (1992) Chilblain lupus erythematosus and lupus pernio – the same entity. Dermatology 185:160.

Paediatrics

CASE 21

A young woman gives birth in midsummer to a daughter. It is immediately evident that the child has severe deformities of both feet (Fig. 21.1).

1. What is the approximate incidence and likely aetiology of this condition?

2. What would be appropriate initial treatment and when should this be started?

3. At what stage would surgery be contemplated?

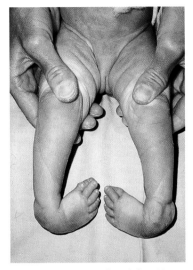

Fig. 21.1 Bilateral foot deformities

Congenital talipes equinovarus

1. Clubfoot has an incidence of approximately 1 in 1000 live births. In the majority the condition is labelled as 'idiopathic', although clubfoot is associated with myelomeningocele, amniotic band syndrome and arthrogryposis. Inheritance is variable but there is probably an underlying single gene anomaly. In the presence of a mutation other factors will predispose the child to contraction of the soft tissues of the foot and abnormal talar development. Deformity may be exacerbated by a reduction in maternal amniotic fluid (oligohydramnios), hence the prevalence of the condition in children born during the summer months, and to disturbances in neuromuscular function producing ipsilateral calf muscle atrophy.

2. The aim of treatment is to reverse the deformity by abducting and externally rotating the mid and forefoot. Whilst doing this, it is important to keep the foot dorsiflexed at the ankle as much as possible to maintain heel alignment and to prevent the development of a 'rocker bottom' deformity of the midfoot. The position is held by applying a dynamic splint as shown (Fig. 21.2).

It is necessary for the physician or a trained therapist to see the child weekly to ensure that the splintage is being satisfactorily applied to maintain the foot in the corrected position. If progressive improvement in the deformity is not evident by 3 months then surgical intervention is required.

3. The optimal timing of surgery and the exact procedures required remain a matter of some debate. The majority of surgeons would probably agree that at least a lengthening of the Achilles tendon should be considered by 9 months at the outside. In Edinburgh, an extended posteromedial release through a transverse Cincinnati incision is favoured (Fig. 21.3),

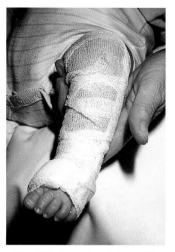

Fig. 21.2 Dynamic splintage with strapping

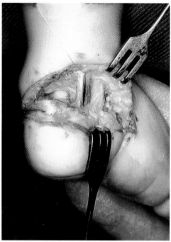

Fig. 21.3 Extended posteromedial release

creating a mobile and plantigrade foot. The foot is immobilized in plaster following surgery to maintain the corrected position.

KEY POINTS

- Clubfoot is common and requires careful early management.
- Splinting will suffice in many instances.
- Surgical intervention should be considered at 3 months.

FURTHER READING

Daniels TR, Alman B, Wedge JH (1999) Congenital clubfoot – paediatric masterclass. Current Orthopaedics 13:229–36.

Macnicol MF (1994) The surgical management of congenital talipes equinovarus (club foot). Current Orthopaedics 8:72–82.

CASE 22

This girl's mother is concerned about her daughter's flat feet (Fig. 22.1). She reports that her shoes develop an abnormal bulging on the medial side of the upper. There are no other symptoms and 'her feet have always been this way'. The heel rise test is shown in Figure 22.2.

1. Describe the clinical features seen in Figure 22.1. Clinically, what do these features indicate?

2. What is the heel rise test (Fig. 22.2), which mechanism is it testing and what does it reveal?

3. What conditions are associated with flat foot in childhood?

4. Why is this parent concerned that her daughter has flat feet?

5. How should this girl's feet be managed?

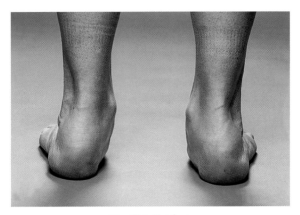

Fig. 22.1 Flat feet

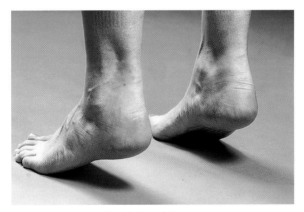

Fig. 22.2 Heel rise test

Flat foot

1. Flat foot (pes planus) is simply a low medial arch. In addition to this, Figure 22.1 demonstrates marked eversion of the hindfoot, Helbing's sign (bowing of the Achilles tendon), prominence of the medial malleolus and abduction of the forefoot. Not only is this foot flat but the rearfoot is in valgus alignment. Excessive subtalar pronation, as occurs for structural foot types such as forefoot varus, causes lowering of the medial arch and so the two conditions are usually associated as pes planovalgus.

2. For the heel rise test, patients are asked to stand on their toes. Normally this will cause the medial longitudinal arch of the foot to increase in height and the calcaneus to invert. With rigidity on toe standing the arch will fail to rise and there will be no inversion of the calcaneus. This test uses Hick's windlass mechanism whereby dorsiflexion of the toes creates tension in the plantar fascia, drawing the forefoot and hindfoot closer. In so doing, this increases the arch and inverts the subtalar joint. An alternative to the heel rise test is Jack's test whereby, on standing, the patient's great toe is dorsiflexed at the MTP joint (Fig. 22.3). This should produce a similar effect to that described above. In this case, arch formation indicated that the flat foot was flexible, excluding a pathological condition such as tarsal coalition from the diagnosis.

3. Flat foot is associated with connective tissue disorders such as Marfan's and Ehler's Danlos syndromes. Neuromuscular conditions such as cerebral palsy and poliomyelitis, rupture of the tibialis posterior tendon and juvenile chronic arthritis may also cause lowering of the medial longitudinal arch. Congenital causes are: tarsal synostosis (case 25) and congenital vertical talus. The latter is a rare but very deforming example of flat foot (Fig. 22.4).

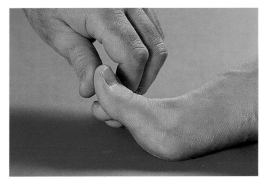

Fig. 22.3 Jack's test

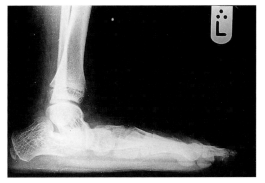

Fig. 22.4 Lateral radiograph: congenital vertical talus

4. At one time pes planus was considered a deformity, and 'fallen arches' were sufficient to prevent recruitment into the army, as they were believed to be detrimental to foot function. The medial longitudinal arch usually increases in height during childhood. Low arches are seen in some races and foot shape is inherited to some extent. Bilateral flat foot in children and adolescents is usually asymptomatic and should not restrict sporting activities. It will not always cause disability during adulthood.

5. A painless flexible flat foot does not warrant surgical intervention. Reassurance should be given to the child and mother that it is a normal variant. If there is pain and it is related to foot function, then custom-made orthoses should be provided to hold the rearfoot in a more neutral alignment and restore stability (Fig. 22.5). However, there is a lack of evidence to suggest that these effect a permanent correction of the deformity, although they can improve foot function.

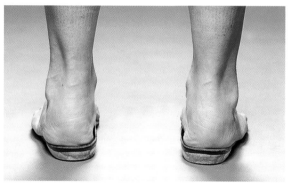

Fig. 22.5 Control of hindfoot malalignment with orthoses

KEY POINTS

- The heel rise test differentiates between a rigid and flexible flat foot.
- Flexible flat foot in children is common and is often a cause of parental concern. It does not usually require treatment.
- Custom-made orthoses should be considered on an individual basis.
- Surgery is never indicated and parents should be reassured.

FURTHER READING

Kitaoka HB, Lou ZP, An KN (1998) Three dimensional analysis of flat foot deformity: cadaver study. Foot and Ankle International 19(7):447–50.

Staheli LT (1999) Planovalgus foot deformity. Journal of the American Podiatric Medical Association 89:94–9.

CASE 23

One of the most common presenting foot abnormalities in children is shown in Figure 23.1.

1. This common digital anomaly is universally described as what? How should management be approached? Is there ever any indication for surgery?

2. How does an overriding toe, as shown in Figure 23.2, differ in aetiology? Which eponym is commonly associated with the correction of this deformity and will surgery be successful?

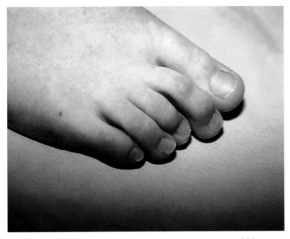

Fig. 23.1 Clawing of the lesser digits in a 14-year-old boy

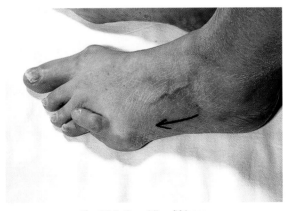

Fig. 23.2 Overriding fifth toe

Claw toe and adductus quinti digiti

1. By far the most common digital anomaly in children is the 'claw' toe. This arises from an imbalance between flexor and extensor muscle power and/or lumbrical muscle weakness. In the absence of a neurological deficit leading to clear evidence of leg muscle weakness, it may be worthwhile attempting to correct the toe clawing by asking the child to perform regular exercises. However, often these are of little value and more definitive surgery is required. The classic operation is that described by Girdlestone (see Taylor, 1951), in which the flexor tendons are detached from the phalanges of the digit and transferred laterally and dorsally to be attached to the extensor tendon.

2. Adductus quinti, or congenital contracture of the fifth toe, is generally a familial deformity. The initial deformity is probably an external rotation of the phalanges of the digit, causing change in the vector of action of the dorsal extensor tendon. The fifth toe is pulled dorsally over the fourth digit and with time the dorsal capsule of the MTP joint contracts.

A variety of surgical procedures have been described to correct this deformity. These range from taking the distal end of the long extensor tendon and passing it under the digit from medial to lateral, as described by Lapidus in 1942, to resection of the base of the proximal phalanx and creation of a syndactyly between the fourth and fifth toes. The commonest procedure is probably that termed Butler's operation, as shown in Figure 23.3. The authors' experience has been that this procedure is fine for young children but it seldom holds the toe in older subjects, as shown in Figure 23.2. Usually an osteotomy of the fifth metatarsal will be required to derotate the toe.

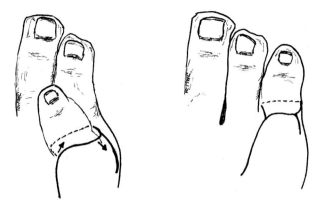

Fig. 23.3 Butler's operation

- Claw toes are generally familial and bilateral.
- Surgery may be required but should be performed before the age of 15 years.
- Overriding of the fifth toe is not easily corrected. The toe often looks short, especially if part of the proximal phalanx is resected.
- Long-term outcomes are not especially good and the patient should be warned that further surgery may be necessary.

FURTHER READING

Cockin J (1968) Butler's operation for an overriding fifth toe. Journal of Bone and Joint Surgery 50-B:78–81.

Taylor RG (1951) The treatment of claw toes by multiple transfers of the flexor into extensor tendons. Journal of Bone and Joint Surgery 33:539–42.

CASE 24

A 9-month-old child was brought by a very concerned mother to the paediatric clinic. Examination of her feet revealed a significant deformity (Fig. 24.1).

1. This deformity is fairly common. What is the primary abnormality and with what other conditions is it associated?

2. Would any form of conservative treatment be appropriate?

3. When will surgery become necessary and what operations have been described?

4. Is a good long-term outcome expected?

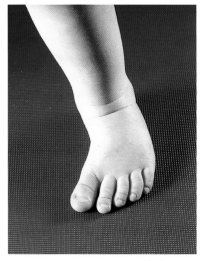

Fig. 24.1 Severe in-toeing in a child of 9 months

Metatarsus adductus

1. The illustration shows metatarsus adductus. In milder forms the soft tissues remain lax and it is generally possible to hold the foot in neutral alignment. In this case virtually no abduction was possible.

The deformity in this instance occurred as an isolated deformity, but metatarsus adductus may be associated with clubfoot and developmental dysplasia of the hip.

2. Advice was sought from a paediatric orthopaedic surgeon and it was recommended that the deformity would correct with time. During the next few months the child was seen regularly by a physiotherapist who progressively stretched out the soft tissues.

3. Forefoot adduction may occur in patients with clubfoot if the midfoot becomes fixed and rigid or if the tibialis anterior muscle is relatively overactive.

The simplest surgical procedure is probably to release the abductor hallucis tendon at the level of the first metatarsal neck, but this procedure is only of value in terms of reducing the duration of conservative therapy. Muscle imbalance must be directly addressed by either split or complete transfer of the tibialis anterior tendon laterally. In the more rigid foot, particularly in older children, a capsular release to mobilize the tarsometatarsal and intermetatarsal joints will be required, or even osteotomies of the metatarsal bases to bring them round into correct alignment.

4. Outcomes from conservative treatment are generally excellent with minimal residual deformity. In this case the child had an entirely normal foot by age 3 years.

KEY POINTS

- Metatarsus adductus may be associated with clubfoot.
- Serial stretching and casting will generally allow remodelling to occur.

FURTHER READING

Berman A, Gartland JJ (1971) Metatarsal osteotomy for the correction of adduction of the fore part of the foot in children. Journal of Bone and Joint Surgery 53-A:498–506.

Heyman CH, Herndon CH, Strong JM (1958) Mobilization of the tarsometatarsal and intermetatarsal joints for the correction of resistant adduction of the fore part of the foot in congenital club-foot or congenital metatarsus varus. Journal of Bone and Joint Surgery 40-A:299–310.

This young lady first presented for treatment of a painful flat left foot aged 12 years. She was offered no treatment at this time. However, she is now 22 years old and her pain has become progressively worse over the past few years. She is unable to pursue her chosen career as a catering manager as this involves being on her feet all day. Instead, she is employed in a video shop where she is able to sit at her work. On examination there appears to be some inversion and eversion of the hindfoot but the heel rise test is negative (Figs 25.1a and b).

1. Diagnose this young lady's foot complaint.

2. Which pathognomonic radiological feature is apparent in Figure 25.2 and why does it occur with this condition?

3. Are there any further investigations you would consider?

4. List the treatment options.

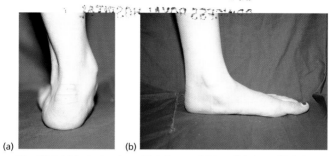

Fig. 25.1 (a) Posterior view of left foot and (b) medial view of left foot

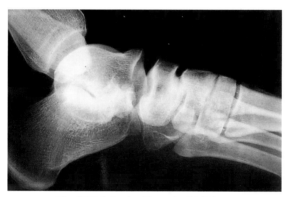

Fig. 25.2 Lateral radiograph of left foot

Talocalcaneal synostosis

1. Talocalcaneal synostosis (peroneal spastic flat foot, tarsal coalition) represents 48% of all tarsal synostoses. Coalition is usually of the medial facet (sustentaculum tali) but involvement of the posterior facet has also been reported. The condition becomes painful in the second decade as the cartilaginous bar ossifies. Examination reveals a loss of subtalar joint movement.

2. X-rays are of limited value although flattening ('beaking') of the head of the talus is pathognomonic and results from abnormal demands on the talonavicular joint for frontal plane motion. The lack of subtalar and midtarsal motion will be countered by increased movement distally, i.e. at the cuneiform metatarsal joints. These are therefore at risk from degenerative arthritis and will be a source of pain.

3. Harris views (ski-jump) projections demonstrate the subtalar joint, but CT scans are probably easier to interpret (Fig. 25.3). In this case bone scans were also taken which revealed hot spots in the midtarsal joints (Fig. 25.4).

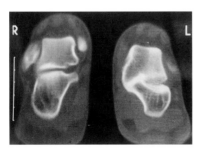

Fig. 25.3 CT image of subtalar joints showing union of the talus and calcaneus at the middle facet of the left sustentaculum talus

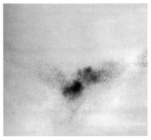

Fig. 25.4 Bone scan showing hot spot in midtarsal joint

4. Although footwear modifications such as medial supports may be helpful, conservative management is not always rewarding. In adolescents, bar excision will diminish symptoms and lessen secondary arthritis. This patient presented too late for this treatment. Although a triple arthrodesis (in effect only an arthrodesis of the talonavicular and calcaneocuboid joints) was successful in the short term, cuneiform-metatarsal arthritis developed later (Fig. 25.5).

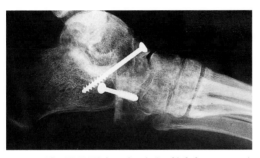

Fig. 25.5 Triple arthrodesis of left foot

KEY POINTS

- Talocalcaneal synostosis presents with a painful flat foot in children and young adults.
- The heel rise test differentiates between a rigid and flexible flat foot.
- 'Beaking' of the talus, apparent on lateral X-rays, is pathognomonic of the condition.
- CT imaging will delineate the extent of tarsal union.
- Early bar excision is recommended.

FURTHER READING

Mann RA, Beaman DN, Horton G (1998) Isolated subtalar arthrodesis. Foot and Ankle International 19:511–19.

Varner KE, Michelson JD (2000) Tarsal coalition in adults. Foot and Ankle International 21:669–72.

CASE 26

These two pictures show very different feet (Figs 26.1 and 26.2).

1. What is the descriptive term used to describe the anomaly shown in Figure 26.1?

2. What are the other characteristics of this familial syndrome?

3. Name the term used to describe shortening of the metatarsals as shown in Figure 26.2.

4. Which metatarsals are most commonly affected and is surgery ever appropriate?

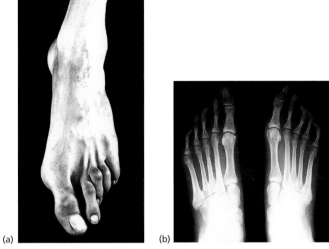

Fig. 26.1 (a) and (b) Long metatarsals

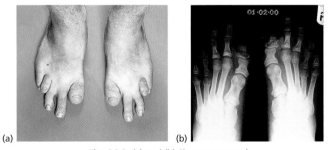

Fig. 26.2 (a) and (b) Short metatarsals

Congenital metatarsal anomalies

1. Figure 26.1 shows the foot of a patient with arachnodactyly (spider fingers) and is virtually pathognomonic of Marfan's syndrome. This condition arises because of a mutation in the *FBN* 1 gene encoding fibrillin 1. It is transmitted as an autosomal dominant trait.

2. The condition is characterized by body disproportion with long limbs, dislocation of the lens, scoliosis, herniae and, in later life, aortic aneurysm. Most of these anomalies are attributable at least in part to ligamentous laxity, as fundamentally the disorder is a collagen disease. Pes plano-valgus is present in approximately 25% of patients. The talus is usually tilted vertically.

Arachnodactyly also occurs in another autosomal dominant condition known as congenital contractural arachnodactyly. Although there is a similar disproportionate body development as in Marfan's syndrome the other features noted do not develop. Joint contracture is present from birth.

3. Shortening of the metatarsals is termed brachymetatarsia (brachymetapody). The patient shown in Figure 26.2 was suffering from spondyloepiphyseal dysplasia tarda, but the condition is also found in several other skeletal dysplasias: for example, achondroplasia, chondroectodermal dysplasia (Ellis–van Creveld syndrome) and pseudohypoparathyroidism. The conditions are frequently autosomal dominant although they may arise as new mutations. An epiphysiodesis of the second and third metatarsal epiphyses, with resection of 1.5 cm of the metatarsal shafts, greatly improved the man's appearance (Fig. 26.3a and b). It was felt that lengthening of the short metatarsals would have been a significant undertaking for someone who was entirely asymptomatic.

4. A short fourth ray alone may also occur, as shown in Figure 26.4. This condition is common in Japanese and is caused by

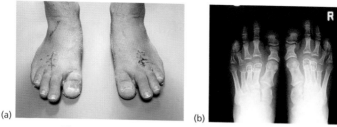

Fig. 26.3 (a) and (b) Postmetatarsal epiphysiodesis

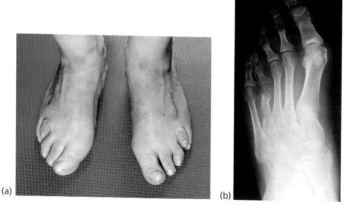

Fig. 26.4 (a) and (b) Congenitally short fourth ray

the premature closure of the epiphyseal plate of the affected metatarsal. The point of metatarsal contact is displaced proximally and the toe offloaded (Fig. 26.5).

Treatment can be quite difficult. Distraction callotasis after metatarsal shaft osteotomy has been advocated, but lengthening may be restricted by the solid anchoring of the distal end of the metatarsal by the transverse metatarsal ligament. Pin tract infections are common and probably a sliding osteotomy with bone graft insertion produces a similar end result, with less discomfort for the patient.

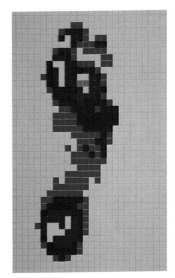

Fig. 26.5 Altered in-shoe contact pressure distribution (Musgrave® system)

KEY POINTS

- A congenital foot deformity is usually part of a generalized syndrome.
- Operative intervention will alter the biomechanics of the foot and it is essential to consider the whole foot rather than simply the deformed part.
- Metatarsal lengthening is limited by the resistance and length of associated neurovascular structures.

FURTHER READING

Choudhury SN, Kitaoka HB, Peterson HA (1997) Metatarsal lengthening: case report and review of literature. Foot and Ankle International 18:739–45.

Lindsey JM, Michelson JD, MacWilliams BA, Sponseller PD, Miller NH (1998) The foot in Marfan syndrome: clinical findings and weight-distribution patterns. Journal of Pediatric Orthopaedics 18:755–9.

The 'at risk' foot

CASE 27

This young nurse presented with a 12-week history of discoloration of her toenail. She first became aware of the lesion when on a 'holiday in the sun'. According to the patient, the lesion has remained static in size since that time.

1. Why is the history of this lesion atypical?

2. What is your provisional diagnosis and which other investigations should be carried out at initial consultation?

3. How are these lesions graded?

4. What do you do now?

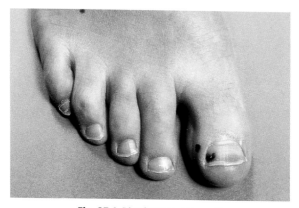

Fig. 27.1 Discoloration of toenail

Melanoma

1. This subungual nail lesion is atypical of trauma. Haematoma normally subside within a few weeks and therefore one would have expected the lesion to have faded. Given the duration and the appearance of the discoloration, further investigation is necessary.

2. It should be an immediate concern that the lesion is a malignant melanoma. Careful examination is required to detect the presence of satellite lesions, and the drainage lymph nodes in the popliteal fossa and groin should be examined for enlargement. Other diagnoses include pyogenic granuloma, onychomycosis, a subungual naevus and a subungual exostosis. A radiograph would immediately exclude the last diagnosis.

Acral lentiginous melanomas make up 10% of UK melanoma cases. They are found on the soles of the feet (Fig. 27.2a and b), the palms of the hands and under the nails. Subungual melanoma was first described by Hutchison in 1883.

3. Melanoma are locally staged according to how thick and deep the lesions are (Breslow grade) and clinically by regional spread (Clark classification) (Table 27.1).

4. If this lesion is shown to be a melanoma then immediate intervention has a bearing on the patient's survival rate. A diagnosis is required urgently. This girl went on to have her nail removed and an excisional biopsy performed within 2 days. The lesion was in fact blood.

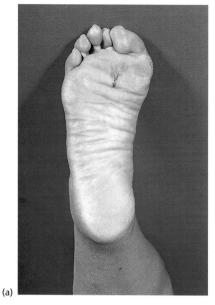

(a)

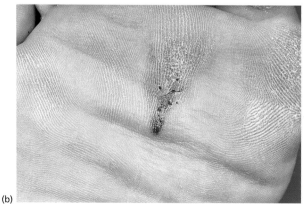

(b)

Fig. 27.2 (a) and (b) Infiltrating melanoma on sole

Table 27.1 Staging of malignant melanoma

	Thickness	Spread	Prognosis
Stage I	<1.5 mm	Upper dermis	Excellent
Stage II	1.5–4 mm	Deep layers of skin – not lymph nodes	May be cured – ?distant metastases
Stage III	>4 mm	Lymph node infiltration. Possible satellite lesions	Better survival if only to local nodes
Stage IV	>4 mm	Distant metastases	<5% 5 year survival

KEY POINTS

- Unusual pigmentation under the nail, especially if of long duration, should be regarded with suspicion.

- Excisional biopsy should be considered to exclude subungual melanoma.

- Acral lentiginous malignant melanoma are often diagnosed late and have a poor prognosis.

FURTHER READING

Bibbo C, Brolin RE, Warren AM, Franklin ID (1994) Current therapy for subungual melanoma of the foot. The Journal of Foot and Ankle Surgery 33:184–93.

Finlay RK, Driscoll DL, Blumenson LE, Karakousis CP (1994) Subungual melanoma: an eighteen year review. Surgery 116:96–100.

Lumsden AB, Clason AE, Lee D, Davies GC (1986) Subungual melanoma of the hallux. A plea for increased awareness. Journal of the Royal College of Surgeons of Edinburgh, February 31:53–5.

Simon H, Etkin MJ, Sodine JE (1999) Well-connected report: melanoma. Nidus Information Services, Inc. www.well-connected.com.

CASE 28

A 75-year-old man presents with skin atrophy and potential ulcer formation under his first and fifth metatarsal heads. The medial hallux sesamoid was excised and a sliding fifth metatarsal osteotomy satisfactorily lessened the pressure on the skin laterally. Unfortunately, the short 1 cm lateral surgical incision would not heal. Blood tests revealed a pancytopenia with features indicative of acute myeloid leukaemia. Within 2 weeks his foot looked as shown in Figure 28.1.

1. What other diagnostic tests should be requested?

2. What options are there for further treatment?

3. If amputation is required, which would be most appropriate for this man?

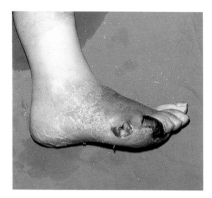

Fig. 28.1 Infected foot

Amputation

1. Clearly the fifth digit is gangrenous and there is significant infection spreading through the soft tissues of the forefoot. Untreated diabetes would be one's first thought, but in this instance there was no evidence of urinary glucose excretion, and a random blood sugar was within normal limits (3–6 mmol/l). The patient's erythrocyte sedimentation rate was, however, elevated and a subsequent blood film revealed a proliferation of myeloblastic precursor cells compatible with an acute myeloid leukaemia.

To establish whether the infection extended into the metatarsals a radiograph was requested and peripheral vascularity assessed by Doppler ultrasound scanning.

2. There was no radiographic evidence of osteomyelitis, but a rampant cellulitis developed despite intravenous antibiotic therapy. Since the average life expectancy for patients with acute myeloid leukaemia is less than 6 months, a below knee amputation was selected as being the most likely method of producing a healed stump and a rapid restoration of mobility. A long posterior flap was cut to take advantage of the better perfusion of the posterior calf skin and facilitate stump healing.

3. A Syme's amputation (Fig. 28.2) was considered, but it was felt that if this were to fail, the patient might spend the majority of his remaining life in hospital. Although it would have been possible to stage the amputation, reducing the risk of spread of infection to the tibia, healing of a Syme's stump is entirely dependent on an adequate blood supply to the heel from the calcaneal branches of the posterior tibial artery. At stage one the foot is removed, leaving the tibial articular cartilage and malleoli, with the wounds closed in standard fashion over a suction drain. Antibiotics can then be instilled

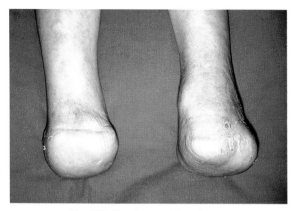

Fig. 28.2 Syme's amputation stumps

locally as a prophylaxis against spread of infection, but most surgeons simply administer these parenterally. At 6 weeks, the malleoli are trimmed through two short incisions and a temporary Syme's prosthesis may be fitted.

A simple fifth ray, a Lisfranc's (tarsometatarsal) or Chopart's (midtarsal) amputation, would have been doomed to failure because of the oedema and swelling of the dorsal foot skin. Similarly, both Boyd's calcaneotibial fusion and Pirogoff's calcaneal section/rotational amputation were discounted as being unnecessarily complicated in this instance. In any case, both the latter two procedures depend on fusion of the calcaneal remnant to the tibia and require at least 8 weeks' stump immobilization in plaster. In contrast, this patient was mobile on a custom prosthesis similar to that shown below within 1 month (Fig. 28.3).

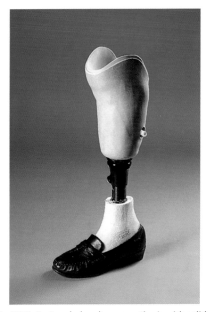

Fig 28.3 Custom below knee prosthesis with solid ankle cushion heel

KEY POINTS

- Always check peripheral circulation and sensation before choosing the resection level.
- Seek the opinion of a second surgeon before proceeding.
- Beware foot equinus following Lisfranc's amputation and equinovalgus after Chopart's amputation.
- A Syme's stump will allow direct end weightbearing.
- Staging a Syme's amputation may prevent spread of sepsis.

FURTHER READING

Burgess EM, Romano RL, Zettl JH, Schrock RD (1971) Amputations of the leg for peripheral vascular insufficiency. Journal of Bone and Joint Surgery 53-A:874–90.

Grady JF, Winters CL (2000) The Boyd amputation as a treatment for osteomyelitis of the foot. Journal of the American Podiatric Medicine Association 90:234–9.

Wagner FW (1977) Amputations of the foot and ankle: current status. Clinical Orthopedics 122:62–9.

CASE 29

A man presents with a painful ulcer on his big toe. His ankle: brachial pressure index (ABPI) is 0.5. A radiograph of his distal phalanx reveals an underlying osteomyelitis (Fig. 29.1a and b).

1. What is the ABPI?

2. How is it measured?

3. Is this an absolute test?

4. What does an ABPI of 0.5 indicate and how should this patient be managed?

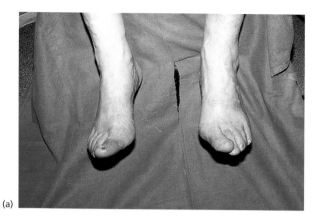

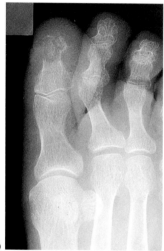

Fig. 29.1 (a) Toe ulcer and (b) radiograph

Ischaemic toe

1. The ABPI is a useful and easily performed clinical technique. It is a sensitive test for arterial insufficiency and provides quantitative information about the arterial supply to the foot.

2. The taking of the ABPI requires measurement of the systolic blood pressure at the arm and ankle. Both values may be obtained with a handheld Doppler ultrasound probe and sphygmomanometer (Fig. 29.2). Systolic pressure at the ankle should equal the central (brachial) pressure, although, in fact, owing to the decrease in calibre of distal vessels, the ankle systolic pressure is normally greater. The pressure index is the ratio of ankle:brachial systolic pressure. Patients with

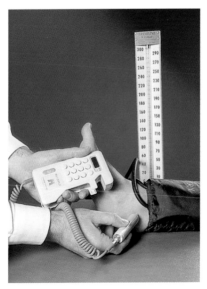

Fig. 29.2 ABPI measurement

Table 29.1 ABPI values, interpretation and implications

ABPI value (x)		Interpretation	Implication
$x \geq 1.3$		Calcification of arteries	Attention required to Doppler wave form. Toe pressures and pole test
$1 \geq x < 1.3$		Normal	
$0.5 \geq x < 1$	Upper limit	Minor disease	Delayed wound healing
	Midrange	Claudication	Significant, symptomatic disease
	Lower limit	Rest pain	Limb at risk from ulceration
$x < 0.5$		Critical limb ischaemia	Vascular surgery

significant atherosclerosis, exhibiting signs of claudication, will have a value of greater than 0.5 but less than 1. A value of less than 0.5 requires urgent vascular intervention (Table 29.1).

3. Although generally a sensitive and reliable measurement, as with most tests, false positive values may occur if there is any arterial calcification (Mönckeberg's sclerosis), in diabetes and in the elderly. Although calcification of the arterial media will not obstruct blood flow, the vessels become less compressible and will lead to a falsely high ABPI. In these cases, attention should be paid to the quality of the Doppler wave form, which should be biphasic or triphasic. A monophasic wave form is indicative of arteriosclerosis. The ABPI can also be used in combination with a subjective evaluation of the circulation such as by Buerger's limb elevation test, in which the leg is raised and noted for pallor. On dependency the return of colour should be brisk. Delayed filling, cyanosis or hyperaemia are indicative of ischaemia. For patients with diabetes mellitus with arterial calcification, the measurement of toe systolic pressures is recommended.

4. The implication of an abnormal ABPI to this man is that his ulcer will not heal until the arterial supply has been improved. The lesion is complicated by underlying osteomyelitis evident in Figure 29.1b for which antibiotics will be ineffective because of the lack of a blood supply. He requires arteriography and probably bypass surgery.

KEY POINTS

- The ABPI is a sensitive measure which is useful to quantify arterial disease.
- Calcification of the arteries will result in a falsely high ABPI.
- Buerger's limb elevation test should be used to complement ABPI measurements.
- Ulcer healing will not take place until a blood supply has been re-established.

FURTHER READING

Donnelly R, Emslie-Smith AM, Gardner ID, Morris AD (2000) Vascular complications of diabetes. British Medical Journal 320:1062–6.

Donnelly R, Hinwood D, London NJM (2000) Non-invasive methods of arterial and venous assessment. British Medical Journal 320:698–701.

Grasty MS (1999) Use of the hand-held Doppler to detect peripheral vascular disease. Supplement to the Diabetic Foot 2:18–21.

Vowden P (1999) Doppler ultrasound in the management of the diabetic foot. Supplement to the Diabetic Foot 2:16–17.

CASE 30

A 54-year-old man was admitted to the trauma unit after his right great toe became swollen. He had no recollection of an injury. An X-ray did not show clear evidence of a lesion but a subsequent MRI revealed significant bone destruction (Fig. 30.1a and b).

1. What are the differential diagnoses of this lesion?

2. Are there any specific attributes that would define a cartilaginous lesion?

3. What treatment is warranted?

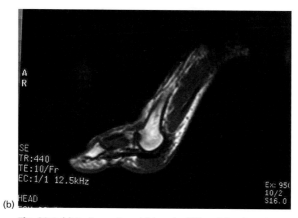

(a)

(b)

Fig. 30.1 (a) Radiograph and (b) sagittal T1-weighted MR image of right great toe

Chondrosarcoma of the great toe

1. The radiograph showed very little, but a well-defined lytic lesion was evident on the MR image shown. Radiolucent swellings that should figure in differential diagnoses would be an intraosseous ganglion, benign tumour of tendon sheath, enchondroma and possibly a secondary deposit. Multiple lesions would be pathognomonic of Ollier's disease or multiple enchondromatosis.

2. Microscopy of a biopsy from the lesion (Fig. 30.2) shows a cellular and lobulated tumour with islands of cartilage filling up the marrow spaces. The nuclei shown are large and both nucleoli and binucleate cells are not difficult to find. Even though there are no mitoses in the section, the cellularity and atypia of the cells make this lesion typical of a chondrosarcoma.

3. After a preliminary biopsy, it is necessary to excise any tumour mass completely, including the biopsy tract. In this instance amputation of the toe was required as, although the tumour was low grade, a wide excision would have left no

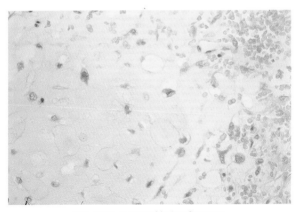

Fig. 30.2 Biopsy of lesion from toe

viable tissue. The patient was subsequently fitted with a total contact insole combined with a toe spacer to compensate for the amputation. It is not likely that any other treatment will be required for a low-grade lesion and the patient's life expectancy should be normal.

KEY POINTS

- Malignant tumours are fairly common in the foot. Beware of melanoma in particular.

- Biopsy may spread a tumour and preclude definitive local resection. Consider referral to a specialist unit if the diagnosis is uncertain.

- Complete excision often necessitates amputation.

- Chemotherapy or radiotherapy may be required.

FURTHER READING

Bovee JV, van der Heul RO, Taminiau AH, Hogendoorn PC (1999) Chondrosarcoma of the phalanx: a locally aggressive lesion with minimal metastatic potential: a report of 35 cases and a review of the literature. Cancer 86:1724–32.

Lo EP, Pollak R, Harvey CK (2000) Chondrosarcoma of the foot. Journal of the American Podiatric Medicine Association 90:203–7.

CASE 31

A 60-year-old man is admitted on 2 January to the medical ward, having been found lying in a disused railway shed. It is noted that his toes are white in colour and somewhat insensitive. Unfortunately, over the next few days the appearances dramatically change (Fig. 31.1a and b).

1. What is the likely cause of this man's foot ischaemia?

2. What factors have led to the appearances found?

3. Is there an urgent need for surgical treatment and what operation would be appropriate?

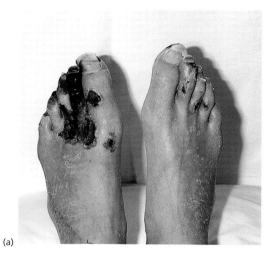

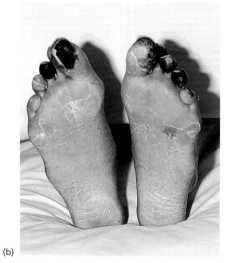

Fig. 31.1 (a) and (b) Toe lesions

Frostbite

1. On arrival in Casualty the patient was found to have a temperature of 35.5°C and it was felt that he had probably been exposed to the elements for some time. Gradual warming soon brought his temperature up to a normal level and restored the colour to his toes, albeit that they became slightly 'mottled'. The initial changes were at first felt to be caused by a generally poor peripheral circulation, but later skin blistering and necrosis were typical of frostbite.

2. The primary aetiological factor in this instance was a prolonged exposure to cold, causing reduced peripheral blood flow by vasoconstriction and increased plasma viscosity. Matters would not have been improved by the patient's consumption of alcohol over New Year, causing dehydration by diuresis. The patient was probably lying immobile for several hours and it was important to exclude a calf or foot compartment syndrome. Either would reduce venous drainage from the periphery and accentuate any ischaemia.

3. Gradually the area of ischaemic tissue demarcated. In areas where small superficial blisters were present a black eschar formed. This separated off in places, leaving a raw area denuded of skin (as shown on the dorsum of the great toe in Figure 31.1). Circumferential injury, however, necessitated amputation.

Theoretically the digits would have spontaneously separated off by 'autoamputation', but this may take in excess of 3 months and it was considered preferable to excise the affected toes surgically as soon as the limitation of the ischaemia was apparent.

Frostbite is a form of gangrene and it is therefore essential to ensure that patients are covered against tetanus. Antibiotic treatment is not required unless a spreading cellulitis develops.

KEY POINTS

- Frostbite should be suspected in patients with hypothermia.
- Check the patient's tetanus immunity.
- Muscle injury with rhabdomyolysis and neural injury may be present.

FURTHER READING

Cauchy E, Marsigny B, Allamel G, Verhellen R, Chetaille E (2000) The value of technetium 99 scintigraphy in the prognosis of amputation in severe frostbite injuries of the extremities: a retrospective study of 92 severe frostbite injuries. Journal of Hand Surgery 25A:969–78.

Pulla RJ, Pickard LJ, Carnett TS (1994) Frostbite: an overview with case presentations. Journal of Foot and Ankle Surgery 33:53–63.

CASE 32

A 55-year-old lady is referred as an emergency. She presents with a painful swollen foot. There is a wound on the sole with a spreading cellulitis apparent along the medial longitudinal arch (Fig. 32.1). She feels generally unwell, having flu-like symptoms.

1. Describe the clinical features apparent in Figure 32.1.

2. This lady does not have the flu but why did she present with these symptoms?

3. Outline the further investigations which were required in this instance.

4. Discuss your immediate management of this patient.

5. What factors have predisposed to this foot condition and how does this influence your management?

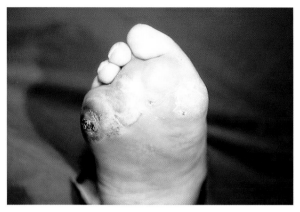

Fig. 32.1 Plantar aspect of foot

Subcutaneous infection

1. The clinical features apparent are cellulitis and lymphangitis. There is a cavity of pus underlying the subcutaneous tissue. The infection is spreading via the lymph vessels in the medial longitudinal arch and is seen 'tracking'. Tissue destruction is also evident.

2. This patient had early signs of septicaemia. Bacteria had spread into the bloodstream (bacteraemia) and are multiplying (septicaemia). Popliteal and inguinal lymph nodes were tender, indicating lymphadenitis.

3. Bacteriological culture identified the precise causative microorganism as *Streptococcus pyogenes* and X-rays excluded osteomyelitis. A neurological assessment was needed to rule out a neuropathy and a vascular assessment to quantify tissue perfusion. Later, foot pressure assessment was carried out to assess plantar pressure distribution.

4. Immediate treatment involved drainage of the lesion (Fig. 32.2). The patient was also provided with strict advice to rest and prescribed erythromycin 500 mg q.d.s. for the spreading infection (Table 32.1).

5. As can be seen from Figure 32.3, and which was confirmed by foot pressure assessment, this lady had pes cavus and needed to wear insoles to deflect pressure from the metatarsal heads. This was followed by the supply of a trauma sandal, adapted to relieve pressure from the area of high loading (Fig. 32.4). On return to clinic 6 weeks later the lesion had healed (Fig. 32.5).

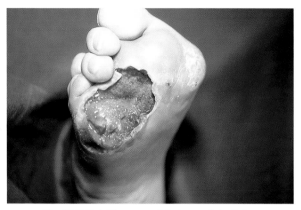

Fig. 32.2 Debridement and drainage of the lesion

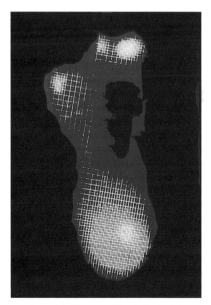

Fig. 32.3 Harris and Beath footprint

Table 32.1 A guide to typical antibiotic therapy for subcutaneous infection

Organism	Description	Antimicrobial therapy – first line drugs
Staphylococcus aureus	Abcesses, yellow pus	Flucloxacillin 500 mg q.d.s., Erythromycin 500 mg q.d.s.
Streptococcus pyogenes	Spreading infection, cellulitis, lymphangitis	Benzylpenicillin 600 mg b.d., Erythromycin 500 mg q.d.s.
Pseudomonas	Thick, foul-smelling green pus	Gentamicin 80 mg t.d.s., Ciprofloxacin 500 mg b.d.
Clostridium	Deep infection, necrosis, gangrene	Benzylpenicillin 600 mg b.d., Metronidazole 400 mg t.d.s.

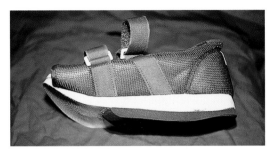

Fig. 32.4 Modified trauma sandal

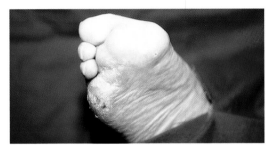

Fig. 32.5 Healed lesion

KEY POINTS

- Treatment of cellulitis demands immediate drainage of the septic lesion and appropriate antibiotic therapy, especially when spreading.
- The causative organism should be identified, as should the precise cause of the lesion.
- Pressure must be removed from areas of high load.

FURTHER READING

Cunha BA 2000 Antibiotic selection for diabetic foot infections: a review. Journal of Foot and Ankle Surgery 39:253–7.

Van der Meer JWM, Koopmans PP, Lutterman JA (1996) Antibiotic therapy in diabetic foot infections. Diabetic Medicine August:48–51.

CASE 33

A 72-year-old lady presents to the clinic concerned that she was walking on the outside of her foot. Clinical examination revealed that she had a chronically discharging leg sinus (Fig. 33.1). This had been diagnosed as a varicose ulcer. A radiograph showed evidence of bone destruction (Fig. 33.2).

1. What is the likely cause of the radiological appearances?

2. What other conditions produce leg ulceration in the elderly?

3. This lady was suffering from no pain yet her ankle progressively adopted a varus deformity. What description is applied to painless arthritis?

4. How would you investigate this lady and what treatment is appropriate?

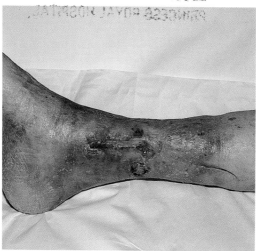

Fig. 33.1 Discharging sinus

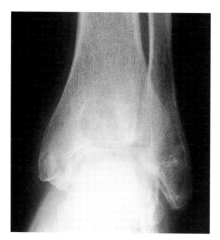

Fig. 33.2 Radiograph of left ankle

Septic arthritis

1. The radiograph shows cystic erosion of the tibial plafond. The presence of peripheral osteophytes suggests that the joint destruction had occurred over a period of time.

2. The appearance might have been caused by rheumatoid disease, but the patient had no other signs of this condition. A copious discharge from, initially, a medial and subsequently a lateral sinus could only be attributable to sepsis.

3. Painless joint arthritis was described in patients with neurosyphilis by Charcot in 1858. Fundamentally, there is an impairment of sensation from the joint receptors, and these changes are characteristically seen in patients with diabetes mellitus, syphilis (tabes dorsalis), syringomyelia and congenital indifference to pain.

4. A swab was sent for culture and sensitivity, but no organisms were grown. Although this might not have been a surprise, as the patient had been on a broad spectrum antibiotic, her erythrocyte sedimentation rate was 86 mm/h.

Drainage, with curettage of any necrotic material, is required to hasten healing. In this instance, however, such a procedure would almost certainly have destroyed any residual capacity that the patient had to weightbear, and the end result would probably have been an amputation.

It was no surprise when the microbiologist finally reported that the infection was due to tuberculosis. The patient was commenced on triple therapy (rifampicin, isoniazid and pyrazinamide) and the discharge diminished dramatically. Eighteen months after starting therapy the radiographic appearance was as shown in Figure 33.3. The patient had no

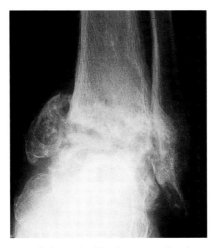

Fig. 33.3 Distal tibia and ankle after 18 months' chemotherapy

pain and was walking in a surgical shoe with a heel flare, albeit using a stick outside. Although the degree of joint subluxation will almost certainly mean that she will require a leg iron in the future, this is clearly a better option than either joint fusion or amputation. A fusion would not only be technically difficult to achieve in the presence of such significant bone destruction, but it is unlikely that the lady would tolerate a further 6–8 weeks in a plaster cast.

KEY POINTS

- Some form of neuropathy must be present in patients with a Charcot joint.
- All patients should be tested for diabetes mellitus.
- Consider tuberculosis as a cause of chronic sepsis.

FURTHER READING

Newman JH (1981) Non-infective disease of the diabetic foot. Journal of Bone and Joint Surgery 63-B:593–6.

Werd MB, Mason EJ, Landsman AS, Hanft JR, Kashuk KB (1994) Peripheral skeletal tuberculosis of the foot. Etiologic review and case study. Journal of the American Podiatric Medicine Association 84:390–8.

Rheumatology

CASE 34

A young woman, in her early twenties, has persistent discomfort in the balls of both feet. Pain and stiffness is worse first thing in the morning. Her symptoms began insidiously, without a history of trauma. On examination, there is obvious swelling of the forefoot and the patient has become aware that her toes appear 'separated' (Fig. 34.1).

1. This girl has an unusual presentation of metatarsalgia. Of what condition should you be suspicious and how frequently are feet affected with this condition?

2. What name is given to separation of the toes as seen in Figure 34.1?

3. Describe the diagnostic X-ray features in Figure 34.2. Is this a common site for this feature?

4. Name the further investigations which are now required.

5. What therapeutic measures should be considered?

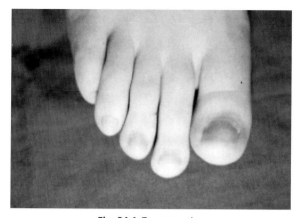

Fig. 34.1 Toe separation

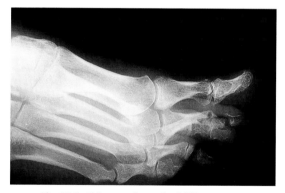

Fig. 34.2 Oblique radiograph of fifth MTP joint

Diagnosis of rheumatoid arthritis

1. In early presentation of rheumatoid arthritis, the feet are involved more frequently than the hands. Patients often complain of 'walking on pebbles'. Further examination will reveal swelling and tenderness in the MTP joints. These are painful when squeezed laterally.

2. Joint effusions can lead to spreading of toes, giving rise to the 'Daylight Sign'. Inflamed and full bursae are likely to be present over the metatarsal heads on the plantar side.

3. X-rays of the feet show diagnostic erosions of the fifth metatarsal head. The metatarsal heads are the most common sites of erosive change, with an order of involvement from metatarsal 5, then 3, 2, 4 and 1. The metatarsal head erodes before the base of the proximal phalanx. The distal IP joints are rarely affected.

4. Investigations should include measurement of erythrocyte sedimentation rate (ESR), tests for rheumatoid factor (latex agglutination/Rose–Waaler tests) and X-rays, which may be unremarkable in early disease.

5. Disease-modifying antirheumatic drugs should be considered to retard the erosive process. Specific foot therapy is aimed at ensuring the patient's footwear is adequately wide at the toe box. Cushioning insoles will also help.

KEY POINTS

- Presentation of pain and swelling in the forefoot without a history of trauma should raise the suspicion of rheumatoid disease, particularly if accompanied by joint pain elsewhere.
- Feet are involved earlier and more frequently than the hands in rheumatoid arthritis.
- MTP joint erosions are diagnostic and indicate the need for second-line drug management.

FURTHER READING

Corbett M, Young A (1988) The Middlesex Hospital prospective study of early rheumatoid disease. British Rheumatology 27(Suppl. II):171–2.

Renton P (1991) Radiology of the foot. In: Disorders of the Foot, 3rd edn. London: Blackwell Scientific Publications, pp. 272–9.

CASE 35

After stepping off a pavement awkwardly a middle-aged doctor suddenly found that her great toe became extremely painful. There was little to observe initially, but during the next week severe swelling developed (Fig. 35.1).

1. Why was the doctor's toe swollen and inflamed? What other conditions may mimic this inflammatory arthropathy and what is its most likely cause?

2. How can the condition be diagnosed in the laboratory? Would a negative blood test exclude the condition?

3. Various treatments are recommended, but which is best? How long should therapy continue?

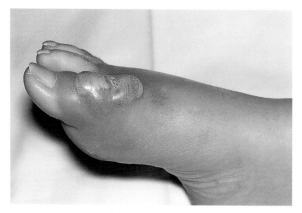

Fig. 35.1 Painful toe

Gout

1. The description is typical of that of a patient with acute tophaceous gout. This condition generally affects men in middle age, but is not uncommon in women after the menopause. In this case swelling of the fingers and presence of gouty tophi are diagnostic (Fig. 35.2).

Chondrocalcinosis, or pseudogout, rarely affects the foot and ankle as calcium pyrophosphate dihydrate crystals are preferentially laid down in articular fibrocartilage or the cartilage at the sites of ligamentous attachments to bone (in the knee, wrist, pubic symphysis and intervertebral discs).

Gout is caused by an elevated serum urate. This is a natural metabolite of the purines guanine and adenine (nucleic acid components), and hence any condition increasing the rate of

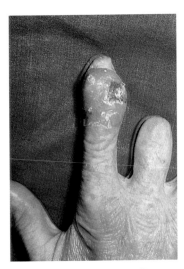

Fig. 35.2 Gouty tophus on finger

purine breakdown, or restricting urate excretion, may precipitate gout. For lack of a more obvious cause, the condition is often attributed to a dietary excess, including high alcohol consumption. It is worthwhile screening patients at their initial attack for any blood disorder causing excessive nucleoprotein production. The practitioner should also ensure that the patient is not on a diuretic altering renal urate filtration.

2. Monosodium urate monohydrate precipitates out to form either an amorphous mass or needle-shaped crystals of 0.2–2 μm in length (Fig. 35.3). A definitive diagnosis will be reached if crystals can be visualized and generally the affected joint must be aspirated. Serum urate levels will not always reflect the severity of the condition. The chance of a patient suffering gout does increase if the urate is elevated above normal, but many patients will maintain normal urate levels outwith their acute attacks.

3. Non-steroidal anti-inflammatory drugs which inhibit cyclo-oxygenase (the enzyme that converts arachidonic acid to prostaglandins) provide analgesia and an anti-inflammatory

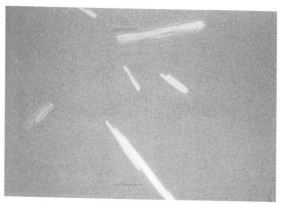

Fig. 35.3 Negatively birefringent urate crystals

effect in acute gout. Salicylate (aspirin) is contraindicated, but colchicine may be considered (0.5 mg 2-hourly until the acute attack settles). An intra-articular corticosteroid injection will sometimes provide temporary symptomatic relief if only one joint is inflamed.

For long-term prevention of recurrent attacks, either uricosuric agents such as probenecid and sulphinpyrazone or the xanthine oxidase inhibitor allopurinol are required. Maintenance doses of allopurinol (200–600 mg daily) are required for life.

KEY POINTS

- Acute gout may be precipitated by trauma or low temperature as these will facilitate crystallization. Peripheral joints are frequently affected.

- Monosodium urate needles are negatively birefringent when viewed under polarized light.

- Allopurinol should not be used as primary treatment for acute gout.

FURTHER READING

Davis JC (1999) A practical approach to gout. Current management of an 'old' disease. Postgraduate Medicine 106:115–16 and 119–23.

Schlesinger N, Baker DG, Schumacher HR (1999) How well have diagnostic tests and therapies for gout been evaluated? Current Opinion in Rheumatology 11:1–5.

CASE 36

Foot problems are only one element of the condition affecting this 25-year-old man. As well as a recent history of plantar and posterior heel pain he also has a history of non-specific urethritis.

1. This condition usually presents as a triad of symptoms. What are they?

2. Who does this syndrome affect, and what is the usual precursor?

3. Enthesitis is a feature of this syndrome. What is it and where does it occur?

4. Arthritis affects mainly which joints and how are they treated?

5. What is the skin lesion shown in Figure 36.2?

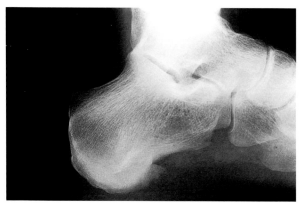

Fig. 36.1 Lateral radiograph of the hindfoot

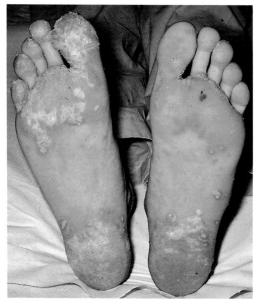

Fig. 36.2 Skin lesions on the sole of the foot

Reiter's syndrome

1. Reiter's syndrome comprises a triad of symptoms: seronegative arthritis, conjunctivitis and non-specific urethritis. Although originally described as this triad, Reiter's disease can still reasonably be diagnosed if one component, usually conjunctivitis, is absent. Other symptoms may also be present, notably balanitis, stomatitis and keratoderma. Some of these give only mild and temporary discomfort.

2. Reiter's syndrome is found in men 13 times more frequently than in women, the age of onset being between 20 and 30 years. It is a reactive arthritis and, in the UK, the commonest precursor is a urethritis. As with the other seronegative arthropathies, there is an association with the HLA-B27 antigen.

3. Enthesopathy, which is an inflammation at the attachment of fascia, ligaments and tendons to bone (entheses) such as the Achilles tendon and plantar fascia, occurs early but is persistent. Sacroiliitis and spondylitis will develop in susceptible individuals. Initially, only soft tissue swelling may be observed radiologically but eventually erosions will be visible and, finally, reactive bone sclerosis. This is characterized in patients with plantar heel pain by the formation of calcaneal spurs that are large and have ill-defined margins (Fig. 36.1). They are described as 'fluffy' in appearance. Erosions also occur at the posterior surface of the calcaneus at the attachment of the Achilles tendon.

4. One joint at a time becomes swollen, with the lower limbs affected more often than the upper. The predilection is for the knees, ankles and toes. The pattern of joint disease is that of a transient, asymmetrical polyarthritis, which develops acutely, subsiding after a few weeks. However, some cases progress to a more chronic relapsing and remitting form of disabling arthritis. Treatment for Reiter's syndrome entails rest for painful joints. Aspiration of swollen joints may be required and corticosteroid injection may be helpful. Non-steroidal anti-inflammatory drugs are generally prescribed, but some patients require sulphasalazine or other disease-modifying antirheumatic drugs.

5. Involvement of the skin of the soles of the feet is termed keratoderma blennorrhagicum. The lesions appear first as brown macules but they rapidly develop into painless, reddened, often confluent raised plaques and pustules. They are similar, both clinically and histologically to the lesions of pustular psoriasis. Toenails become dystrophic which can cause them to separate off, with regrowth after 3–6 months. Keratoderma is helped with the application of hydrocortisone cream.

KEY POINTS

- Reiter's syndrome is a triad of seronegative arthritis, conjunctivitis and non-specific urethritis.
- Enthesopathy is a common feature and can affect the plantar fascia and insertion of the Achilles tendon.
- Keratoderma blennorrhagicum affects the soles of the feet.

FURTHER READING

Conska GW (1987) Reiter's syndrome. Update, 15 December:1284–94.

Tozzi MA, Stamm R, Bigelli A, Hart D (1981) Reiter's syndrome: a review and case report. Journal of the American Podiatric Medicine Association 71:418–22.

CASE 37

The fingernails hold the key to the diagnosis of this man's painful foot. He is 32 years old and presents in clinic with an acutely painful and swollen right second toe (Fig. 37.1). He also complains of pain in his right heel and ring finger of his right hand. On close examination there is pitting of his fingernails (Fig. 37.2).

1. Which radiological features are evident on inspection of the radiograph in Figure 37.3?

2. Given the clinical and radiological presentation, which condition is this?

3. Which digit is most commonly affected and which other joints may be involved?

4. What might a radiograph of the heel reveal?

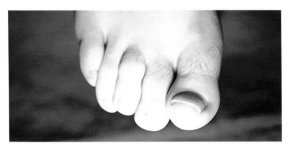

Fig. 37.1 Sausage toe

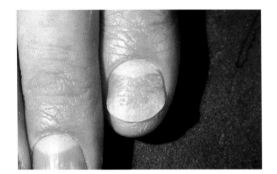

Fig. 37.2 Pitting of the fingernails

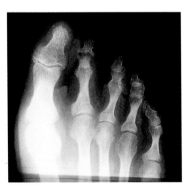

Fig. 37.3 Anteroposterior radiograph
of the forefoot

Psoriatic arthritis

1. The radiograph in Figure 37.3 reveals intra-articular erosions at the second DIP joint and fusion at the second PIP joint. The fifth DIP joint is not apparent, which may be the result of joint fusion or, more likely, biphalangism.

2. Psoriatic arthritis is a seronegative joint disease mainly affecting the small peripheral joints and the spine (spondyloarthropathy). The patient may have skin lesions over the extensor aspects of the elbows and knees, but skin involvement may be minimal or hidden, such as when the scalp is affected. The pattern of joint disease illustrated in this case is described as an asymmetrical oligoarthritis involving scattered small joints, giving rise to 'sausage' digits (Fig. 37.4). Psoriatic arthritis may also present as a type that is indistinguishable from rheumatoid arthritis, or as the rare but very destructive arthritis mutilans.

3. Psoriatic arthritis most commonly affects the great toe, but radiological changes may be seen at any of the IP joints.

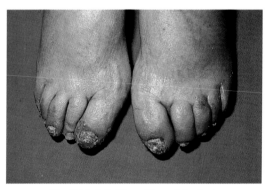

Fig. 37.4 Arthritis mutilans of the foot

There is a tendency for the condition to involve the feet before the hands. More severe disease brings about 'pencil and cup' deformities. Joint ankylosis may occur secondary to a periostitis that causes new bone to be laid down along the joint margins. This is the primary cause of sacroiliitis.

4. Inflammation at the origin of the plantar fascia commonly presents as a painful heel. Radiographs often reveal large heel spurs that have irregular and ill-defined cortical margins. The enthesopathy can be accompanied by insertional Achilles tendinitis.

KEY POINTS

- Psoriatic arthritis affects the joints of the hands, feet and spine.
- Skin involvement may be hidden.
- Psoriatic arthritis can present as a very destructive arthritis mutilans.
- Heel spurs are large with an irregular cortical outline.

FURTHER READING

Gerster JC, Piccinin P (1984) Enthesopathy of the heels in juvenile onset seronegative B27 positive spondyloarthropathy. Journal of Rheumatology 12:310–14.

Renton P (1991) Radiology of the foot. In: Disorders of the Foot, 3rd edn. London: Blackwell Scientific Publications, pp. 272–9.

CASE 38

The foot is involved in most patients with rheumatoid arthritis. An elderly lady with established rheumatoid disease repeatedly attends the podiatry clinic (Fig. 38.1a and b).

1. Describe the pathological changes that have taken place to result in this forefoot deformity.

2. How is the rest of the foot affected with rheumatoid arthritis?

3. How should this patient be managed?

4. Is there a role for surgery here?

5. Which non-articular features of rheumatoid arthritis are sometimes found in the foot and lower limb?

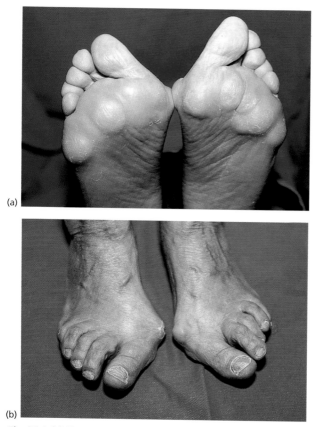

(a)

(b)

Fig. 38.1 (a) Plantar aspect and (b) dorsal aspect of rheumatoid forefoot

Therapy of rheumatoid arthritis

1. In established rheumatoid disease, there are a number of classical features. There is a high prevalence of hallux valgus (90%); the joints become subluxed and the toes become clawed with fixed flexion deformity of the joints. The plantar fibrofatty pad, which is intended to protect the metatarsal heads, is pulled distally and exposes the metatarsal heads (Fig. 38.2). The prominence of the metatarsal heads in turn leads to high pressures, resultant bursae and plantar callosities. A combination of increased local pressure and relative ischaemia creates a risk of ulceration and secondary infection. Figure 38.3 shows osteoporosis, bone destruction and deformity.

2. There is a low or absent medial longitudinal arch and the foot as a whole is in valgus alignment (pes plano valgus). This valgus attitude is caused by the collapse of the subtalar joint. Synovitis, articular erosion and stretching of the ligaments have allowed the talar head to adduct and plantarflex with resultant bulging of the foot medially. This process of deformity is exacerbated by valgus alignment of the knee. The calcaneus is in a fixed valgus alignment and the forefoot is abducted. The extremely valgus heel can impinge on the

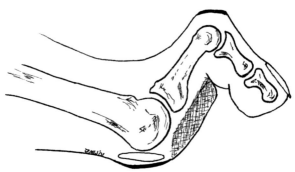

Fig. 38.2 Prolapse of the metatarsal heads in rheumatoid arthritis

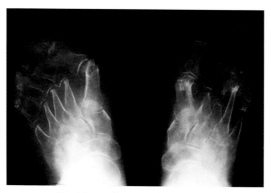

Fig. 38.3 Radiograph of the forefoot

fibula. Excessive pronation places a strain on tibialis posterior (stance phase inverter of the foot) which often ruptures, exacerbating the valgus alignment. The patient's gait tends to be antalgic and apropulsive, with a prolonged double support stance phase. The ankle joint is less frequently involved in rheumatoid arthritis.

3. Soft insoles relieve pressure from the painful metatarsal heads (Fig. 38.4). Orthoses are valuable to improve the alignment of the foot and to relieve forefoot pressure. Bespoke or semi-bespoke footwear is important to accommodate hallux valgus and digital deformities. These can be modified with a Thomas heel and medial heel flare to create medial stability, which has been lost with progressive valgus alignment of the foot.

4. Surgical management is aimed at relieving forefoot pressure usually by some form of excisional or replacement arthroplasty of the forefoot. Additional operations for the rheumatoid foot include triple arthrodesis of the hindfoot to produce a more plantigrade foot, arthrodesis of the ankle, tibialis posterior repair and selective toe surgery.

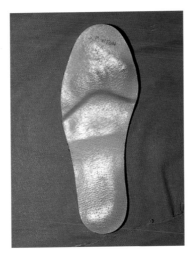

Fig. 38.4 Soft insole

5. Vasculitis and rheumatoid nodules occur in patients with high titres of rheumatoid factor and severe erosive disease. Vasculitic ulcers tend to be deep with sharp margins ('punched out'). They occur anywhere on the leg and foot, but are more common on the lower leg (Fig. 38.5). These

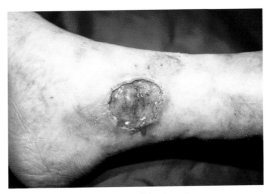

Fig. 38.5 Vasculitic ulceration

ulcers are painful and difficult to treat. Lesions occur during the active stage of the disease and require disease-modifying antirheumatic drugs. Subcutaneous nodules are present in 20% of patients with rheumatoid arthritis. These feel firm, non-tender and are freely movable, although they can be attached to deeper structures. In the foot they occur over the MTP joints, around the Achilles tendon and on the extensor surface of the toes.

KEY POINTS

- The forefoot is the source of great discomfort to patients with rheumatoid arthritis.
- The metatarsal heads become prominent and are subjected to excessive pressure which increases the risk of ulceration.
- Palliative insoles and suitable footwear are essential.
- Vasculitis and nodules occur in aggressive disease.

FURTHER READING

Cawley MID (1987) Vasculitis and ulceration in rheumatic diseases of the foot. Baillière's Clinical Rheumatology 1(1):315–32.

Cracchiolo A (1993) The rheumatoid foot and ankle: pathology and treatment. The Foot 3:126–34.

King J, Burke D, Freeman MAR (1978) The incidence of pain in the rheumatoid hindfoot and the significance of calcaneo-fibular impingement. International Orthopaedics 2:255–7.

Sibbitt WL, Williams RC (1982) Cutaneous manifestations of rheumatoid arthritis. International Journal of Dermatology 21:563–71.

Stockley I, Betts RP, Rowley D, Getty C, Duckworth T (1990) The importance of the valgus hindfoot in forefoot surgery in rheumatoid arthritis. Journal of Bone and Joint Surgery 72-B:705–8.

Neurology

CASE 39

This patient regularly has to remove her shoe while shopping. She is a 45-year-old female research worker who presents with a sharp, shooting pain in the ball of her left foot and toes. The pain began as a burning, tingling sensation, which is now more intense and neuralgic in nature. She is only able to walk short distances. Relief of pain can be aided by massaging her foot or manipulating her toes. On examination, there is a sensory deficit in the region demonstrated in Figure 39.1. Pain is exacerbated by lateral compression of her forefoot (Fig. 39.2).

1. Name this condition and state the group of patients most commonly affected by it.

2. Which test is being carried out in Figure 39.2 and precisely where would you expect to localize pain?

3. Name additional investigations that are helpful in confirming a diagnosis.

4. Discuss the aetiology of this condition.

5. Outline a treatment plan for this patient.

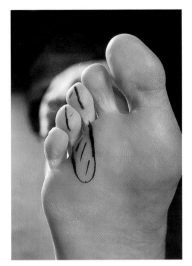

Fig. 39.1 Area of sensory deficit affecting the toes

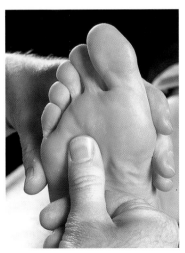

Fig. 39.2 Clinical examination of the foot

Morton's neuroma

1. Morton's neuroma is a common, paroxysmal neuralgia affecting the web spaces of the toes. Pain arises from a pathological plantar digital nerve as it divides to supply the adjacent sides of the toes it innervates. The mean age of presentation is between the years of 45 and 50 and women are affected overwhelmingly. Bilateral presentation is relatively uncommon, as is the occurrence of more than one lesion in the same foot.

2. Using a thumb, firm pressure applied to the affected web space will elicit focal tenderness which may be exacerbated by simultaneously compressing the metatarsal heads together (Fig. 39.2). This may be accompanied by a painful 'Mulder's click'. The third web space is most frequently involved, followed by the second. It is extremely rare for symptoms to occur in either the first or fourth web spaces. The exact site of tenderness is located to a point between and just anterior to the heads of the two adjacent metatarsals. Other clinical signs and symptoms are summarized in Table 39.1.

3. Over the past few years high resolution, diagnostic ultrasonography has been routinely used to detect neuroma. A typical sonographic appearance is that of a hypoechoic mass (varying in density from the surrounding tissue), orientated parallel to the long axis of the metatarsals (Fig. 39.3). Although recent studies question the validity of ultrasound scans in relation to histopathology of the nerve, our approach is to confirm a swelling on the nerve with ultrasound before operation.

4. Histological changes are consistent with an entrapment neuropathy of the plantar digital nerve. Constrictive footwear is implicated as the main causative factor in compressing the nerve. This is substantiated by the relief of pain found on

Table 39.1 Summary of the clinical signs and symptoms of Morton's neuroma

Subjective symptoms	Objective symptoms
• Sharp, lancing or cramp-like pain (often likened to a burning hot needle) • Pain only on walking • Patient has to stop walking • Patient has to rest until pain goes (relief aided by removing shoes and massaging toes) • Pins and needles or numbness experienced between toes	• Pain located in second or third web space (elicited with plantar pressure and exacerbated by lateral compression) • Painful Mulder's click present • Loss of sharp sensation between toes • Injection of local anaesthetic temporarily ameliorates pain

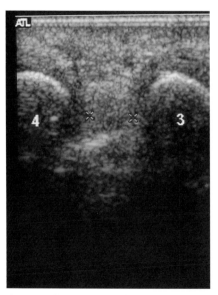

Fig. 39.3 Ultrasound scan of the intermetatarsal spaces showing a swelling on the plantar digital nerve to the third and fourth toes

shoe removal and the higher occurrence of the condition in women. Pain may be compounded by shearing stresses in a hypermobile forefoot, giving rise to an MTP bursitis that indirectly compresses the nerve.

5. Conservative management starts with advice to the patient to change the style of their shoes. Broad, lace-up shoes are to be recommended and slip-on court shoes avoided. Insoles can only be considered if the footwear will accommodate them, or they will worsen the problem. Insoles such as a teardrop pad with its apex sited between the metatarsals will spread the metatarsals. Orthoses can be used to reduce forefoot hypermobility.

An injection of corticosteroid is the third line of treatment and anecdotally is beneficial in about 50% of patients (see clinical tip below). If this fails then the neuroma is easily resected through the sole of the foot (Fig. 39.4). Although a dorsal incision avoids the risk of a scar that can be troublesome on weightbearing, it is necessary to divide the intermetatarsal ligament to reach the neuroma and

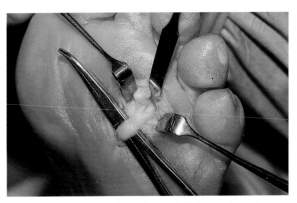

Fig. 39.4 Excision of the plantar digital nerve through a plantar incision

occasionally this will produce splaying of the digits after surgery. A four-stage treatment plan is summarized below:

1. Patient education regarding footwear modifications and palliative padding or insoles.
2. Biomechanical assessment with a view to providing orthoses, if appropriate.
3. Injection of hydrocortisone.
4. Surgical excision of nerve.

Clinical tip: corticosteroid injection for Morton's neuroma

Injection of corticosteroid is a standard treatment for Morton's neuroma.

Solution/volume:	Methyl prednisolone 0.5 ml (20 mg) and lignocaine hydrochloride 1 ml (2%)
Needle:	A 25-gauge (blue) needle or 27-gauge (long) needle is ideal
Technique of injection:	Locate the painful intermetatarsal space, invariably the second or third. Identify the metatarsal heads and, from the dorsum, introduce the needle just proximal to the level of the metatarsal heads (Fig. 39.5). Penetrate until resistance of the plantar skin is met. Withdraw the needle about 0.5 cm, aspirating to avoid intravascular injection, and then inject half the volume of contents of the syringe. Withdraw the needle a further 0.5 cm and inject the remainder.

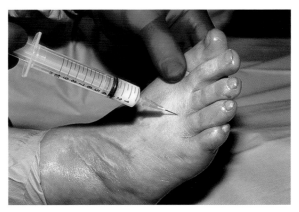

Fig. 39.5 Injection of corticosteroid for Morton's neuroma

KEY POINTS

- Morton's neuroma is common, affecting mainly the third web space.
- Pain is characteristically paroxysmal and limits walking.
- Footwear is the dominant causative factor.
- Management is directed at advice on footwear, use of insoles and corticosteroid injections.
- Excision of the nerve remains the mainstay of treatment.

FURTHER READING

Bourke G, Owen J, Machet D (1994) Histological comparison of the third interdigital nerve in patients with Morton's metatarsalgia and control patients. Australian and New Zealand Journal of Surgery 64:421–4.

Morscher E, Ulrich J, Dick W (2000) Morton's intermetatarsal neuroma: morphology and histological substrate. Foot and Ankle International 21:558–62.

Okafor B, Shergill G, Angel J (1997) Treatment of Morton's neuroma by neurolysis. Foot and Ankle International 18:284–7.

Oliver TB, Beggs I (1998) Ultrasound in the assessment of metatarsalgia: a surgical and histological correlation. Clinical Radiology 53:287–9.

Thomson CE, Campbell R, Wood A, Rendall GC (2001) Disorders of the adult foot. In: Lorimer et al: Neale's Common Foot Disorders, 6th edn. Edinburgh: Churchill Livingstone, pp. 158–66.

CASE 40

Many people have high foot arches yet remain entirely asymptomatic. They only present to podiatry or orthopaedic clinics when they develop clawing of the toes or hard calluses on their soles. In this case a lady in her mid-fifties presented to the clinic complaining that she continually walked on the outer border of her foot. A radiograph confirmed that she had marked heel varus (Fig. 40.1).

The lady reported that in 1954 she had surgery to her great toe and the following photographs were retrieved from the hospital archives (Fig. 40.2a–c).

1. What is the likely aetiology of this patient's long-standing cavoid foot?

2. How is the degree of structural deformity quantified?

3. What operations had been performed in 1954?

4. What procedure corrected the hindfoot varus?

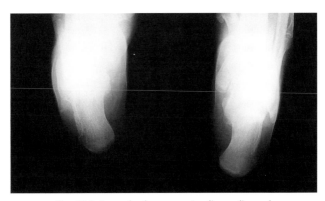

Fig. 40.1 Severe heel varus on standing radiograph

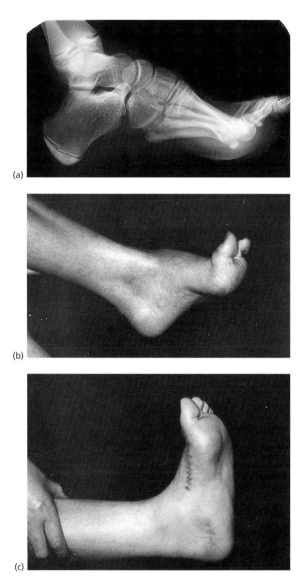

Fig. 40.2 (a)–(c) Clinical appearance in 1954

Poliomyelitis

1. In many parts of the world poliomyelitis still remains the commonest cause of pes cavus, although similar changes may be evident in patients with cerebral palsy, some forms of muscular dystrophy and in Charcot–Marie–Tooth disease. Muscle imbalance may be extremely subtle yet can lead to significant deformity. In polio there is usually weakness of the dorsiflexor muscles and some calf contracture, although the reverse can occur leading to calcaneocavus. Frequently, callosities develop under the metatarsal heads, along the outer margin of the foot and across the dorsum of the PIP joints at the site of toe hammering.

2. Pes cavus is quantified by measurement of the first metatarsal–calcaneal angle on a standard weightbearing lateral foot radiograph. This angle will be less than 140°, as in this instance (Fig. 40.3). Although the heel may lie in a neutral position, a structural varus deformity of the forefoot progressively develops with tightening of the plantar fascia. The tendency for the patient to bear weight on the outer border of the foot leads to progressive forefoot adduction.

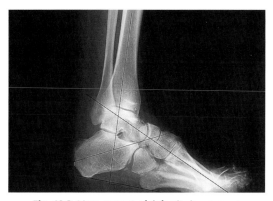

Fig. 40.3 Measurement of defomity in pes cavus

The ultimate aim of surgery for pes cavus is to obtain a plantigrade foot. If the tibioplantar angle exceeds 120°, then forefoot cavus will not be corrected by a basal metatarsal or tarsometatarsal wedge excision without creating a rocker bottom foot and a triple arthrodesis is generally required.

3. At the age of 11 years, this patient had a Steindler release of the plantar fascia from her heel, with a 70% correction of the cavus. Subsequently, extensor hallucis longus was transferred to the neck of the first metatarsal (Jones transfer). The surgeon chose not to fuse the IP joint of the great toe. Tibialis anterior function was noted to be strong and further surgery, such as transfer of extensor digitorum longus tendons to the cuneiforms (Hibb's procedure), was not required.

4. The primary residual deformity at the patient's recent presentation was the severe varus of her heel on her left side. She had no subtalar pain and a lateral closing wedge osteotomy of the calcaneus (Dwyer's osteotomy) produced an extremely satisfactory end result (Fig. 40.4a and b).

In this case the patient's forefoot cavus was not especially severe and a more distal dorsal tarsal wedge osteotomy (or Japas' V osteotomy) was not required.

KEY POINTS

- Pes cavus is common and is frequently asymptomatic.
- Surgery should be undertaken in the teenage years if possible.
- A calcaneal osteotomy will be required to correct heel varus.

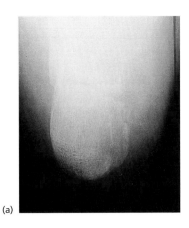

(a)

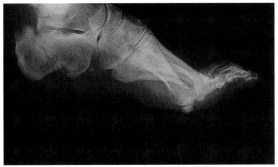

(b)

Fig 40.4 (a) and (b) Correction of heel varus by lateral closing wedge osteotomy

FURTHER READING

Cole WH (1940) The treatment of claw-foot. Journal of Bone and Joint Surgery 22:895–908.

Dwyer FC (1959) Osteotomy of the calcaneum for pes cavus. Journal of Bone and Joint Surgery 41-B:80–6.

Jahss MH (1983) Evaluation of the cavus foot for orthopaedic treatment. Clinical Orthopaedics 181:52–63.

Japas LM (1968) Surgical treatment of pes cavus by tarsal V-osteotomy; preliminary report. Journal of Bone and Joint Surgery 50-A:927–44.

CASE 41

A 45-year-old man has type I insulin-dependent diabetes mellitus. He presents with a painless plantar ulcer (Fig. 41.1).

1. What are the main factors that lead to foot ulceration in diabetes mellitus?

2. What investigations are appropriate?

3. How would you manage this patient?

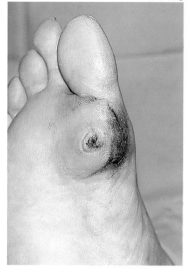

Fig. 41.1 Plantar ulceration

Diabetic neuropathic ulcer

1. The principal factors that lead to ulceration in patients with diabetes are neuropathy, ischaemia and abnormal plantar pressure loading.

2. The priority for assessment of this patient is to establish which of the following prevails.

Neuropathy

Motor neuropathy. Gross inspection of the foot may reveal an abnormal arch and clawing of the toes, indicating intrinsic muscle wastage. Structural changes affect foot function and altered loading, and this is reflected in the presence of plantar calluses.

Sensory neuropathy. In the presence of plantar ulceration there will be decreased perception of pain across the forefoot and this patient demonstrated a loss of sharp/blunt discrimination. Semiquantitative assessment of light touch can be obtained using a 10 g Semmes–Weinstein monofilament. Loss of vibration can be performed using a 128 Hz tuning fork. To give a quantitative assessment a neurothesiometer may be used.

Patients with diabetes mellitus typically present with sensory loss in a 'glove and stocking' distribution. Joint proprioception is absent and consequently the body does not adapt to excessive stresses placed across the foot and ankle joints. Articular cartilage destruction and bone erosion swiftly follow, leading to destroyed insensate Charcot joints (Fig. 41.2a and b). It is important, therefore, to X-ray the entire foot and ankle. Radiological features will include both destructive and hypertrophic changes. Often, there will be marked loss of the affected joint spaces, with fragmentation and resorption of subchondral bone and osteophyte formation.

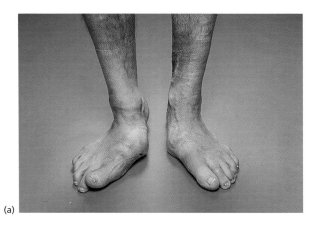

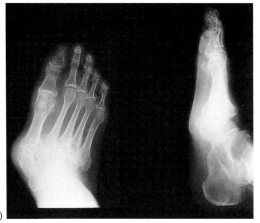

Fig. 41.2 (a) Clinical appearance and (b) radiograph of Charcot joints

Autonomic neuropathy. This is apparent if the skin is dry and flaky, and perhaps also by distension of the dorsal veins, which is a sign of arteriovenous shunting which can lead to changes in blood flow and result in a net loss of bone contributing to joint neuropathy.

Arteriopathy

Gangrene is indicative of ischaemia and is illustrated in Figure 41.3. Thrombosis of the digital arteries has led to gangrene of the toe. It is often secondary to infection, which in this case involves both the soft tissues and phalanx. If the lesion is dry then the digit can be left to autoamputate. In this case the lesion was malodorous and required amputation and antibiotics.

Assessment of arterial disease predicts the outcome of ulcer healing. If the foot is found to be sufficiently ischaemic then the ulcer will not heal. Ankle:brachial pressure indices are important in assessment but the clinician should be mindful of the caveat of a raised index due to Mönckeberg's sclerosis (arteriolar calcification) when, due to arteriovenous shunting, blood short-circuits the toes. The latter is detectable with a hand-held Doppler ultrasound probe as a loud, monotone signal. Digital systolic pressures can be measured with a toe cuff (Fig. 41.4). A normal toe:brachial index is >0.7.

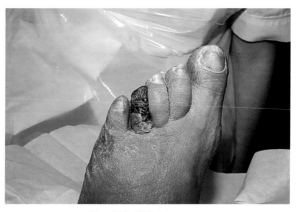

Fig. 41.3 Digital gangrene

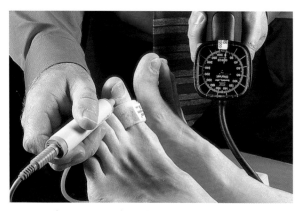

Fig. 41.4 Digital systolic pressure measurement

Infection

Cellulitis will be accompanied by inflammation, although if the blood supply is compromised then this may not be obvious. Deep probing of the wound is required to exclude deep infection that will require surgical drainage and excision of any necrotic tissue. Bone destruction, sequestrum formation and subperiosteal new bone are radiological features of osteomyelitis.

3. The clinician should have two aims. Firstly, it is essential to prevent spread of infection from the ulcer and it should be immediately debrided of all necrotic tissue and a broad-spectrum antibiotic prescribed. Later, to encourage vascularity, the wound may be dressed with a hydrogel, hydrocolloid or alginate as appropriate. Secondly, to prevent recurrent ulcer formation, and indeed generally before healing can be established at all, the plantar pressure must be redistributed. In this case an Aircast® Walker (Fig. 41.5), was used, but a total contact plaster shoe would probably have worked just as well. In the longer term, diabetic insoles and footwear (Fig. 41.6), together with regular visits to a podiatrist, are essential.

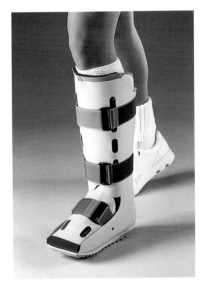

Fig. 41.5 Aircast® Pneumatic Walker

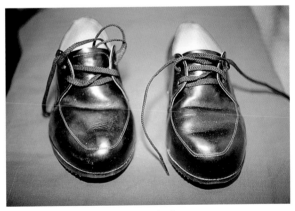

Fig. 41.6 Bespoke footwear

KEY POINTS

- Neuropathic joints lead to gross deformity in the diabetic foot.

- The insensate diabetic foot is at risk from ulceration from increased plantar pressures. This, combined with peripheral vascular disease, leads to poor wound healing and increases the risk of infection.

- Assessment of diabetic ulceration must include assessment of infection, neuropathy and arteriopathy.

- Healing of neuropathic ulcers is established by relief of high pressures and careful wound care.

FURTHER READING

Baker N, Rayman G (1999) Clinical evaluation of Doppler signals. The Diabetic Foot 2:19–25.

Laing P (2000) Surgical management of the Charcot foot. The Diabetic Foot 3:44–8.

Mason J, Keefe CO, Hutchinson A, McIntosh A, Young R, Booth A (1999) A systematic review of foot ulcer in patients with Type 2 diabetes mellitus. I: prevention. Diabetic Medicine 16:801–12.

Mason J, Keefe CO, Hutchinson A, McIntosh A, Young R, Booth A (1999) A systematic review of foot ulcer in patients with Type 2 diabetes mellitus. II: treatment. Diabetic Medicine 16:889–909.

Spencer S (2001) Pressure relieving interventions for preventing and treating diabetic foot ulcers (Cochrane Review). In: The Cochrane Library Issue 2, Oxford: Update software.

CASE 42

A young boy presents to the clinic after his mother noted that his right foot had a higher arch than his left (Fig. 42.1). She stated that he had never played sport, as he was rather 'clumsy' and uncoordinated with poor balance. Examination revealed that his calves were thin, especially in comparison with his thighs where his muscles were clearly well developed. In addition, he had slight weakness of intrinsic muscle power in both hands.

1. Why should this boy's father be examined?

2. What tests are valuable in establishing his diagnosis?

3. If he had presented at 40 years of age, would his diagnosis have been different?

4. Will any form of therapy be beneficial and what other deformities may develop?

5. Will the boy have a normal life expectancy?

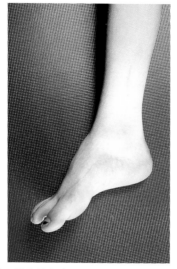

Fig. 42.1 Right leg wasting and cavoid foot

Peroneal muscular atrophy

1. The patient presents with a progressive wasting disorder causing weakness of the peroneal muscles and a cavoid foot. At this age of onset the condition is probably classical peroneal muscular atrophy (Charcot–Marie–Tooth disease), although several other similar conditions have been described. Charcot–Marie–Tooth is an autosomal dominant condition and therefore a familial trait would be expected.

2. Generally, the peripheral nerves are palpable and, on electrophysiological testing, there will be marked slowing of motor and sensory nerve conduction velocities. Muscle biopsy will show grouping of fibres by type, and evidence of denervation and reinnervation. Roussy–Lévy syndrome is similar but patients are aware of a tremor. The lesser types of hereditary motor and sensory neuropathies (types III–VII) are quite rare. The foot disorders are shown in Table 42.1.

3. In later life, patients present with the neurological variant (type II) of the disease. This also has an autosomal dominant inheritance. Although peripheral weakness can be greater, the hands are less often involved. Normal, or near normal, nerve conduction velocities are generally observed on testing and the nerves are not hypertrophic.

4. An orthosis is often required to prevent foot inversion. In mild cases an extended Thomas lateral heel flare on the shoe may suffice, but more severely affected patients will require an ankle–foot orthosis or caliper (Fig. 42.2). A triple arthrodesis is usually necessary eventually to maintain a plantigrade foot. Hand tendon transfers and correction of any scoliosis may also be required in severe cases.

5. Life expectancy should be normal.

Table 42.1 The hereditary motor sensory neuropathies

Type	Disease	Age	Inheritance	Foot deformity
I	Charcot–Marie–Tooth	<20 years	Dominant	Pes cavus
II	Charcot–Marie–Tooth	Middle age	Dominant	Pes cavus
III	Dejerine–Sottas	Infancy	Recessive	Talipes equinovarus
IV	Refsum	0–30 years	Recessive	Pes cavus. Anomalies of metatarsal length
V		10 years onwards	Recessive	Achilles tendon contracture
VI	+ Optic atrophy		Uncertain	Pes cavus
VII	+ Retinitis pigmentosa		Recessive	Pes cavus

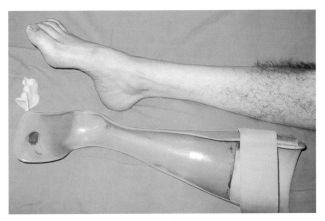

Fig. 42.2 Ankle–foot orthosis

KEY POINTS

- There are two common types of peroneal muscular atrophy with onset at different ages.
- An orthosis is almost always required to prevent foot inversion.
- A triple arthrodesis is frequently necessary in later life.

FURTHER READING

Dyck PJ, Lambert EH (1996) Lower motor and primary sensory neuron diseases with peroneal muscular atrophy. Part I. Neurologic, genetic and electrophysiologic findings in hereditary polyneuropathies. Archives of Neurology 18:603–18.

Dyck PJ, Lambert EH (1996) Lower motor and primary sensory neuron diseases with peroneal muscular atrophy. Part II. Neurologic, genetic, and electrophysiologic findings in various neuronal degenerations. Archives of Neurology 18:619–25.

Trauma

CASE 43

A 36-year-old window cleaner presents, having slipped 20 feet off a ladder. He landed awkwardly on his left heel, which immediately became extremely swollen. In casualty a radiograph confirmed that he had fractured his calcaneus (Fig. 43.1).

1. What is the most common mechanism of injury and what other fractures might have been sustained when the patient fell?

2. How are calcaneal fractures classified? What methods might be used to ascertain the exact type of injury?

3. What treatment is appropriate for this patient?

4. Will the long-term prognosis be favourable?

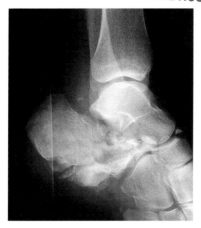

Fig. 43.1 Fracture of calcaneus

Fracture of the calcaneus

1. Most frequently patients land on a pronated foot, destroying their medial longitudinal arch and forcing the heel into valgus. The peroneal tendons will generally be held in their groove on an intact lateral wall. Vertical shear force will produce an initial fracture line (described by Palmer, Fig. 43.2), splitting the bone into two parts: an anteromedial fragment including the sustentaculum tali and a posterolateral fragment including the calcaneal tuberosity. Further fractures propagate according to the force and exact direction of injury.

Calcaneal fractures are bilateral in 5–10% of patients, associated with other lower limb fractures in up to 25% and with a lumbar spinal fracture in 10%.

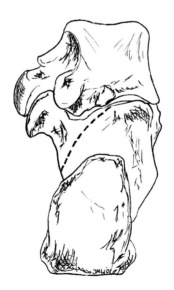

Fig. 43.2 Primary vertical shear fracture

2. In terms of future disability, fractures with an intra-articular extension will generally have a poorer prognosis than those that do not. Calcaneal fractures are no exception and early radiological classifications (by Böhler and Essex-Lopresti) subdivided the fracture types into two primary groups, according to whether the posterior subtalar articular surface was involved.

Extra-articular fractures (25% of the total) of the upper or lower border of the body, tuberosity, anterior process and sustentaculum tali generally have a good clinical prognosis, with many patients able to return to work within 6 months.

Transarticular fractures are less easily classified. Essex-Lopresti considered two primary subgroups. In the first type a downward force causes heel eversion at the subtalar joint and a 'tongue-type' fracture (Fig. 43.3a and b). In the second a shear force typically fractures off the sustentaculum tali, depressing the centrolateral articular segment into the calcaneal body, as shown in Figures 43.1 and 43.4.

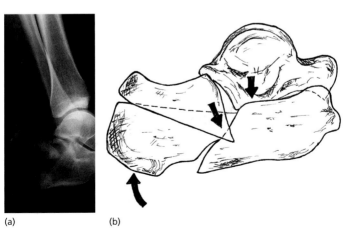

(a)   (b)

Fig. 43.3 (a) and (b) Tongue-type fracture

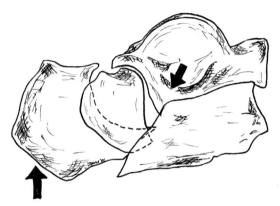

Fig. 43.4 Joint depression fracture

To ascertain the exact pattern of injury further imaging by tomography, CT or MR may be required (Fig. 43.5).

3. Heel fractures are invariably accompanied by massive soft tissue contusion, and immediate high elevation of the injured foot is essential (Fig. 43.6). In this case, the patient's fracture was also extremely comminuted and it was felt that the joint surface was destroyed beyond salvage. However, as noted on the CT image, the heel was excessively splayed. A closed

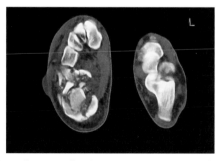

Fig. 43.5 Coronal CT scans showing severe comminution and primary shear

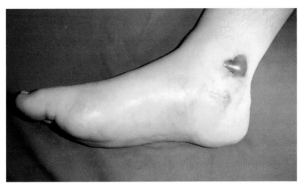

Fig. 43.6 Inner sole bruising (Oxford sign) with fracture blistering

manipulation was performed under general anaesthetic, once the initial swelling was down, and a well-padded plaster cast applied. After a further period as an in-patient with his foot elevated, the patient was allowed to mobilize on crutches without weightbearing. The cast was retained for 6 weeks. Despite intensive physiotherapy during the next 3 months the joint progressively ankylosed (Fig. 43.7).

If surgery had been possible then the essence of treatment would have been to realign the subtalar joint, restoring Böhler's calcaneotuber joint angle (the angle between the

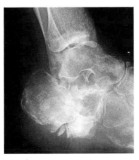

Fig. 43.7 Subtalar joint destruction

superior surfaces of the calcaneus) to that of the opposite foot (normal range 25–40°). A tongue-type fracture may simply be displaced back into position using a lever, sometimes termed a Gissane spike, inserted posteriorly into the bone. The fracture can be held with a couple of screws or staples (Fig. 43.8).

Open reduction and fixation is generally required for joint depression fractures. Often bone graft must be inserted to buttress the joint and the fracture is then usually held by a plate (Fig. 43.9).

4. Rehabilitation after a calcaneal fracture is prolonged and the average time off work for patients in most reported series is about 6 months. Function is impaired by any ankle, subtalar or midtarsal joint stiffness.

Heel cushioning may help relieve pain caused by disruption of the heel fat pad, but if bone spurs on the sole or lateral calcaneal wall cause localized pressure or tendon impingement, respectively, then bone resection may be necessary. A few patients, such as illustrated, will still complain of unremitting pain 12 months after injury. A formal subtalar fusion may then be the only option.

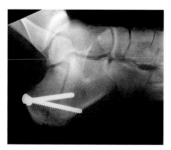

Fig. 43.8 Fracture stabilization with interfragmentary screws

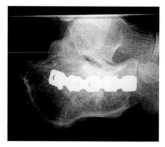

Fig. 43.9 Lateral wall buttress plate

KEY POINTS

- Bruising on the inner aspect of the sole suggests a heel fracture – 'the Oxford sign'.
- High elevation of the foot will lessen initial discomfort.
- Restoration of subtalar joint congruity is the key to a good clinical outcome.
- Bone grafting may be required to buttress the joint surface.
- Physiotherapy is essential to prevent stiffness.

FURTHER READING

Essex-Lopresti P (1952) The mechanism, reduction technique and results in fractures of the os calcis. British Journal of Surgery 39:395–419.

Stephenson JR (1987) Treatment of displaced intra-articular fractures of the calcaneus using medial and lateral approaches, internal fixation and early motion. Journal of Bone and Joint Surgery 69-A:115–30.

CASE 44

Despite braking as hard as possible, a 22-year-old student was unable to prevent his Alfa Romeo crashing at speed into an oncoming car. He suffered the compound fracture shown (Fig. 44.1).

1. What exactly has caused this injury?

2. Who described these injuries and what type would this be?

3. Is subchondral bone atrophy significant? When is avascular necrosis likely to be evident?

4. Would there be merit in any form of hindfoot arthrodesis? If so, which and when?

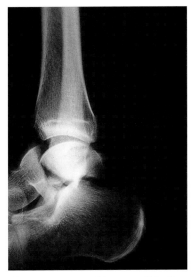

Fig. 44.1 Compound fracture of hindfoot

Fracture dislocations of the talus

1. It was always assumed that talar neck fractures were caused by the leading edge of the tibia striking the talus when the foot was excessively and forcibly dorsiflexed. Cadaveric modelling, however, suggests that it is more likely that it is simply the midfoot which is hyperextended on the talus, when the leg and foot are outstretched, i.e. the hindfoot is held rigid by a taut Achilles tendon. Such a position typically occurs in a 'head-on' motor vehicle accident when the foot is pushed upwards by the pedals or, as originally described, by a similar mechanism in a light aircraft crash, 'the aviator's fracture'. Recently, a boy of 9 years was admitted after sledging backwards (Fig. 44.2a and b).

2. Hawkins classified injuries of the talar neck into three groups: type I, undisplaced talar neck fracture; type II, fracture of the talus with subluxation of the subtalar joint; type III, fracture of the talus with dislocation of the bone from both the subtalar and ankle joints. A fourth type has since been added to take into account any associated subluxation or dislocation of the talar head off the navicular bone.

The 22-year-old patient described suffered a type II injury. He was treated by wound debridement and stabilization of the fracture with two lagged cortical screws (Fig. 44.3).

3. Although fracture malunion can occur, leading to impingement of the dorsal bone surface on the margin of the distal tibia on dorsiflexion, we have found that the protuberant lip of bone is generally resectable and patients regain normal foot function. In stark contrast, avascular necrosis develops slowly and it may be up to 2 years before the condition becomes clinically evident. Avascular necrosis occurs in up to 50% of type II injuries, however treated. Subchondral bone atrophy (Hawkins' sign), seen

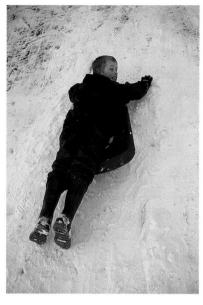

(a)

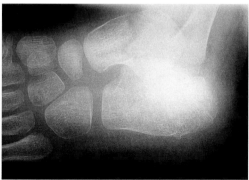

(b)

Fig. 44.2 (a) and (b) Talar neck fracture in a sledger

approximately 6 weeks after a talar fracture is said to be a good prognostic indicator. The sign is probably a reflection of increased localized bone vascularity and healing.

239

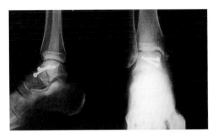

Fig 44.3 Talar neck fracture held by screws

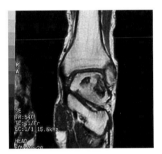

Fig. 44.4 MR image of avascular
necrosis of talus

4. Once avascular necrosis sets in, or if there is significant articular damage to either the subtalar or ankle joints, then further surgery is generally required. Unfortunately, the loss of talar height will mitigate against a successful single joint arthrodesis.

Pantalar hindfoot arthrodesis may be the only viable option and some leg length discrepancy from shortening is an inevitable result. Most trauma surgeons would not consider astragalectomy (talus excision).

KEY POINTS

- Talar neck fractures were classified by Hawkins.
- Avascular necrosis may not be evident for up to 2 years.
- Hawkins' sign indicates a favourable prognosis.

FURTHER READING

Hawkins L (1970) Fractures of the neck of the talus. Journal of Bone and Joint Surgery 52-A:991–1002.

Metzger MJ, Levin JS, Clancy JT (1999) Talar neck fractures and rates of avascular necrosis. Journal of Foot and Ankle Surgery 38:154–62.

CASE 45

Abnormal foot mechanics have an influence on the function of the entire lower limb. A 35-year-old male dentist road runs about 20 miles a week. He would like to increase his running distance but is prevented from doing so because he suffers from pain in both shins. His pain is in the lower third of the inside of his legs. He is noted to have bilateral tibia varum (Fig. 45.1) and a pronated foot on standing. The lateral borders of his shoes show excessive wear (Fig. 45.2). A fellow runner has informed him that his problem is 'shin splints' and that he requires 'orthotics'.

1. Is the fellow runner correct in his diagnosis?

2. Discuss the possible causes of this patient's pain.

3. What is the association between tibia varum and development of shin splints?

4. Will 'orthotics' help this patient?

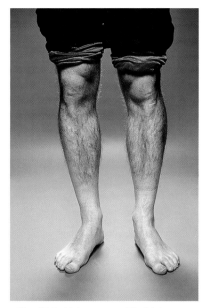

Fig. 45.1 Male runner with tibial varum and pronated feet

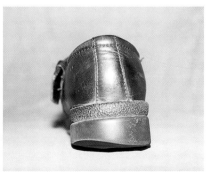

Fig. 45.2 Heel of left shoe showing excessive lateral wear

Shin splints

1. 'Shin splints' is a term used by athletes that encompasses a variety of causes for pain in the leg including soft tissue injuries, periostitis, compartment syndrome and stress fractures. In this sense, the fellow runner is correct in his assessment. However the precise location and nature of the pain has to be determined before therapy can be applied. Shin splints may affect the anterior, lateral and posterior-medial compartments of the leg.

2. Possible causes:

Periostitis. Periostitis of the muscle attachment of tibialis posterior is due to excessive foot pronation. Tibialis posterior acts mainly to decelerate pronation and also to re-establish supination of the subtalar joint towards the end of the mid-stance phase of gait. Prolonged or excessive subtalar joint pronation will create a strain on the attachment of tibialis posterior to the tibia.

Stress fracture of the tibia. Abnormal repetitive loads on bone, in this case tibia varum, mean that available pronation is used to make the foot plantigrade and therefore it loses shock absorption. Patients present with localized pain, swelling and inflammation. Suspected fractures are confirmed by X-ray. Treatment is normally a short period of rest and avoidance of exercise before a gradual return to activity.

Compartment syndrome. Exercise-induced compartment syndrome results from an increase in muscle bulk within tight fascial compartments, causing ischaemia of the enclosed muscles and nerves. Athletes present with aching or cramping in the leg as exercise progresses. Symptoms become progressively more severe and paraesthesia may be experienced in the posterior tibial nerve distribution.

3. Symptoms are related to the patient's tibia varum, because the varus alignment of the leg and foot requires compensatory subtalar joint pronation in order to make the foot plantigrade.

4. The use of an orthosis is dependent on the cause. This patient was diagnosed as having a periostitis of the tibia at the attachment of tibialis posterior muscle and therefore an orthosis was successful in limiting foot pronation. Figure 45.3 shows a custom-made orthosis consisting of a medial heel wedge designed to reduce abnormal foot pronation.

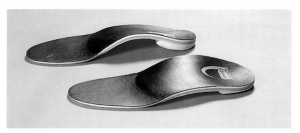

Fig. 45.3 In-shoe orthoses with a medial heel wedge

KEY POINTS

- Shin splints are an overuse injury of the leg.
- They may occur as a result of excessive subtalar joint pronation.
- Orthoses improve symptoms when the cause is a soft tissue injury.
- Other causes of shin splints are stress fracture of the tibia and compartment syndrome.

FURTHER READING

Rzonca EC, Baylis WJ (1988) Common sports injuries to the foot and leg. Clinics in Podiatric Medicine and Surgery 5(3):591–611.

Subotnick SI (1975) Shin splint syndrome of the lower extremity. In: Podiatric Sports Medicine. New York: Futura Publishing Company Incorporated, ch 8, pp 79–81.

CASE 46

A 60-year-old lady presents to the Accident Department complaining that she had slipped on a stairway in a shopping mall. She complained of an extremely sore left heel. The Casualty Officer found that she retained a full range of ankle movement but that she was unable to stand on her toes. An X-ray of her ankle was normal.

An ankle sprain was diagnosed and the patient's ankle was immobilized in a short-leg weight-bearing plaster. The cast was removed 2 weeks later.

The lady's pain persisted throughout the next 3 months. She finally sought a further opinion from her GP who found a lump at the insertion of her Achilles tendon. Surgical exploration revealed what is shown in Figure 46.1.

1. What clinical test should the Casualty Officer have performed?

2. If the diagnosis had been correctly made, would plaster immobilization of the ankle have been appropriate treatment?

3. How can a chronically ruptured tendon be reconstituted and what complications may arise?

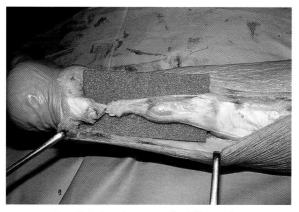

Fig. 46.1 Chronic rupture of Achilles tendon

Chronic rupture of Achilles tendon

1. Simmond's (or Thompson's) test is performed with the patient kneeling on the side of an examination couch. Absence of plantar flexion of the left foot, as shown when this patient was examined, indicated that her Achilles tendon was ruptured (Fig. 46.2).

2. In young patients, in whom one would expect good healing, conservative treatment is perfectly reasonable. The foot should be immobilized in full equinus for 4 weeks, semi-equinus for 4 weeks and then in a 90° cast for a further fortnight. The patient is then encouraged to wear a shoe with a 2 cm heel raise for a further 3 months. In this case, the patient was slightly older than average and, if early diagnosis had been made, then either an open or semi-open (percutaneous) repair method would have been appropriate.

3. If a tear is long-standing, the tendon ends cannot easily be approximated and some form of tendon augmentation is

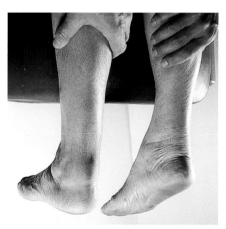

Fig. 46.2 Simmond's test for Achilles tendon rupture (positive on left)

required. The authors' preference is to slide the tendon distally by a V-Y plasty at the musculotendinous junction (Fig. 46.3) or, if some tissue can be stretched across the gap, to use flexor hallucis longus (FHL) tendon as an active augment (Fig. 46.4). Tendon atrophy may occur, with subsequent wound breakdown, when either plantaris or a long strip of the median raphe of gastrocnemius has been turned down across the gap, as shown in Figure 46.5. Presumably this is because the tendon slip is virtually avascular. Subsequent wound salvage may require sophisticated plastic surgery using either a fascial flap, or a micro-vascular free flap, transferred from the forearm or anterolateral thigh.

This patient still had persistent pain and discomfort at her heel 9 months after surgery, with some residual calf muscle weakness. This is not an uncommon finding even if a ruptured tendon is treated acutely.

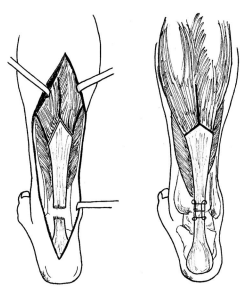

Fig. 46.3 Myofascial slide (V-Y plasty)

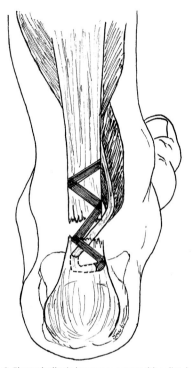

Fig. 46.4 Flexor hallucis longus augment (the distal end of FHL is sutured to flexor digitorum longus)

KEY POINTS

- Achilles tendon rupture is most likely with oblique loading (for example, on heel adduction) of a maximally contracted muscle.

- Conservative management may lead to slower restoration of normal function but postoperative complications are avoided.

- Repair of a chronic rupture generally requires tendon augmentation. A myofascial slide is recommended.

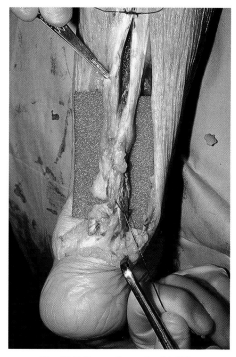

Fig. 46.5 Bosworth repair of Achilles
tendon (not recommended)

FURTHER READING

Abraham E, Pankovich AM (1975) Neglected rupture of the Achilles tendon.
  Journal of Bone and Joint Surgery 57-A:253–6.

Maffulli N (1999) Rupture of the Achilles tendon. Current concepts review.
  Journal of Bone and Joint Surgery 81-A:1019–36.

Wapner KL, Hecht PJ, Mills RH (1995) Reconstruction of neglected Achilles
  tendon injury. Orthopedic Clinics of North America 26:249–63.

Webb JM, Bannister GC (1999) Percutaneous repair of the ruptured tendon
  Achillis. Journal of Bone and Joint Surgery 81-B:877–80.

CASE 47

An overweight, 65-year-old lady reports a constant ache in her foot arches, extending into her calf. She was also aware of an event in which her feet 'gave way' and her 'arches dropped'. Since this event her ache had lessened but she now complains of a weakness in her feet and a lack of spring in her step. This patient has also noted that she has needed a larger size of shoes (see Figs 47.1 and 47.2).

1. What is the most likely diagnosis for this patient's complaint?

2. Explain why she now requires a larger shoe size?

3. Which clinical feature is exhibited in Figure 47.2?

4. What further clinical examination should be carried out?

5. When is surgery indicated for this condition?

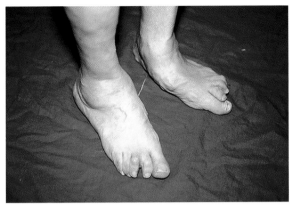

Fig. 47.1 Clinical appearance of patient's feet, medial aspect

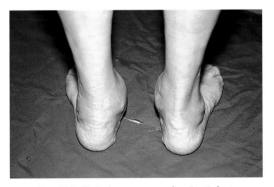

Fig. 47.2 Clinical appearance of patient's feet, posterior aspect

Tibialis posterior rupture

1. Tibialis posterior rupture is the most likely diagnosis. It is a degenerative disorder seen in elderly females with pes planovalgus.

2. Patients may report an increase in shoe size as the feet excessively pronate and the feet consequently elongate.

3. The 'too many toes' sign which occurs with excessive foot pronation results in abduction of the forefoot on the hindfoot (Fig. 47.2).

4. Further examination requires the patient to stand on one foot and then tiptoe. Most patients with a rupture of the tibialis posterior tendon will find this difficult, although it is still possible with the aid of the other posterior calf muscles. To distinguish tibialis posterior dysfunction, the test should be taken a step further and the patient asked to transfer their weight from the outside of their foot to the inside. Dysfunction of the tendon is apparent when the patient fails to perform this action, instead swaying at the hips in an attempt to transfer load on the foot. The patient will also be unable to counteract forcible dorsiflexion and eversion of their foot by the examiner, when non-weightbearing.

5. Direct tendon repair is generally possible if the tendon has recently ruptured. If, however, the tear is long-standing, a graft will be required to bridge the gap. Unfortunately, many patients are seen far too late even for such a reconstruction. The presence of hindfoot arthritis will mitigate against success and the only surgical solution is then a triple arthrodesis to correct the hindfoot malalignment.

If the patient is unfit for surgery, her footwear should be modified to prevent hindfoot pronation. Simplest is probably the

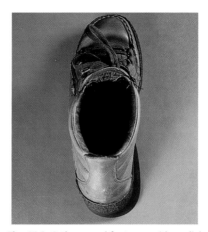

Fig. 47.3 Orthoses and footwear with medial heel flare for tibialis posterior dysfunction

addition of a medial heel flare (Fig. 47.3), but a Thomas style heel will also help if coupled with a supportive in-shoe wedge.

KEY POINTS

- Tibialis posterior dysfunction is generally seen as a degenerative disorder.
- Patients are typically elderly overweight women.
- Orthoses are designed to prevent foot pronation.
- Surgery is an option for acute injuries.

FURTHER READING

Holmes GB, Mann RA (1992) Possible etiological factors associated with rupture of the posterior tibial tendon. Foot and Ankle International 13:70–9.

Johnson KA, Strom DE (1989) Tibialis posterior tendon dysfunction. Clinical Orthopedics 239:196–206.

Mosier SM, Lucas DR, Pomeroy G, Manoli A (1998) Pathology of the posterior tibial tendon in posterior tibial tendon insufficiency. Foot and Ankle International 19:520–4.

CASE 48

A 35-year-old woman jumped down approximately 2 metres off a wall while out hill-walking. She was subsequently brought to Casualty where she was found to have an extremely bruised forefoot. The radiograph is shown opposite (Fig. 48.1).

1. What injury is this?

2. How are these metatarsal dislocations classified?

3. What is the key to fracture reduction and stability?

4. Can a reasonable functional result be expected?

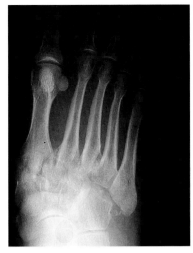

Fig. 48.1 Right foot following injury

Fracture dislocations of the tarsometatarsal joints

1. The radiograph shows a fracture dislocation of the forefoot through Lisfranc's joint. Lisfranc (1790–1847) was a French surgeon of renown who was best known for his work on rectal cancer. His name has been accorded to the ligament anchoring the base of the second metatarsal to the medial cuneiform. This ligament effectively holds the base of the second metatarsal into its recess between the cuneiforms. There is no ligament between the first and second metatarsal bases. Various modifications of an early classification of fracture dislocations by Quénu & Kuss (1909) have been put forward. Most were derived from a consideration of the direction of imparted force to the forefoot (Fig. 48.2). There may be total incongruity of the joint in any plane (a), a partial displacement with only part of the joint incongruent following a lateral (b) or medial force (c) and, finally, the result of a divergent force that may again be subdivided according to whether there is partial or total joint displacement (d).

2. The key to reduction is the placement of the base of the second metatarsal back into its recess. It may be possible to manage this by closed reduction under general anaesthesia, but often the reduction will not be stable and fixation using multiple K-wires or screws is required (Fig. 48.3). The tibialis anterior tendon may become trapped between the medial and intermediate cuneiform bones blocking reduction of the first metatarsal. Open reduction is then essential. Care should be taken that local bleeding and general contusion of the soft tissues has not led to a dorsal foot compartment syndrome. It is generally advisable to release any fascia that appears excessively tight. Patients are kept non-weightbearing for 6 weeks following surgery.

3. The outcome is very much dependent on accurate diagnosis and treatment. Care should be taken in patients

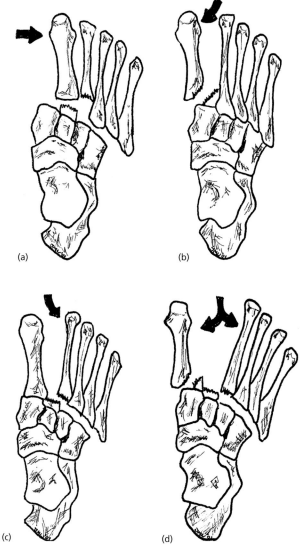

(a)

(b)

(c)

(d)

Fig. 48.2 Lisfranc fracture dislocations of the forefoot

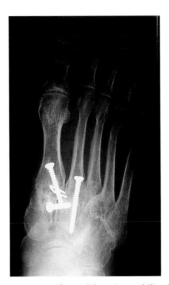

Fig. 48.3 Lisfranc dislocation stabilized with interfragmentary screws

with multiple injuries to ensure that a Lisfranc dislocation is not missed. The only sign present initially may be a bruising under the skin of the midfoot (Lisfranc's sign) and it is only later on weightbearing, that a 'gap' indicative of divergence of the first and second metatarsals is evident. On occasion, patients may not provide a history of acute trauma, as the deformity can be the end result of repetitive injury, especially if a patient has peripheral neuropathy.

4. Unfortunately, even with expeditious treatment, patients often complain of long-term pain in the forefoot. As seen in Figure 48.1, many patients have fractures extending into at least one of the midfoot joints and the end result may be progressive osteoarthritis and residual joint displacement. Most patients will end up with a flat foot deformity and walk taking an increased load on their hindfoot.

KEY POINTS

- Lisfranc dislocation may be missed – look for plantar bruising.
- The base of the second metatarsal must sit in its recess.
- Stabilization is generally required.
- Long-term stiffness is common.

FURTHER READING

Buzzard BM, Briggs PJ (1998) Surgical management of acute tarsometatarsal fracture dislocation in the adult. Clinical Orthopedics 353:125–33.

Hardcastle PH, Reschauer R, Kutscha-Lissberg E, Schoffmann W (1982) Injuries to the tarsometatarsal joint. Incidence, classification and treatment. Journal of Bone and Joint Surgery 64-B:349–56.

CASE 49

Sesamoid bones can be the source of pathology. This 29-year-old schoolteacher was playing tennis in September. She described jumping for a smash, landing heavily and immediately feeling pain in her big toe joint. It is now February and her pain has not improved. It is worse on walking and relieved by rest. Examination reveals a high arched foot, a plantarflexed first ray and tenderness in the region of her medial sesamoid bone. Radiographs of her first MTP joint and sesamoids are as shown (Fig. 49.1a and b).

1. Has this tennis player fractured her sesamoid bone or is this a bipartite sesamoid? Which is more likely?

2. What other conditions affect the sesamoids?

3. What is the treatment for sesamoid pain?

4. When is surgery of the sesamoid bones considered?

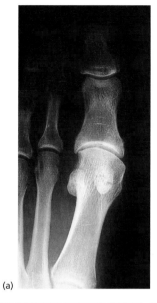

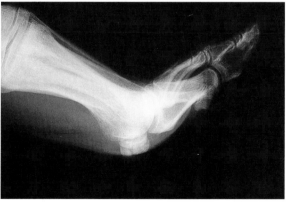

(a)

(b)

Fig. 49.1 (a) AP radiographs (b) lateral radiographs of sesamoid bones

Sesamoiditis

1. True fracture of the sesamoids is rare and fractures are more likely to be stress-related. Fractures should be differentiated from partite sesamoids, which are commonplace, occurring in approximately 25% of individuals. In 80% the medial sesamoid is affected and 90% are bilateral. A fractured sesamoid is not corticated at its fracture line and is only slightly longer than its normal neighbours. A bipartite or tripartite sesamoid is usually larger than a single sesamoid and the partite segments are oval with smooth concave/convex opposing edges (Fig. 49.2). Although partite sesamoids are much more common, given the history, this patient's symptoms and the radiological appearances, it would appear that she has a fracture of her medial sesamoid.

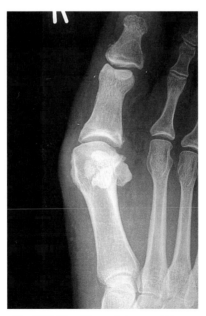

Fig. 49.2 Tripartite medial sesamoid bone

2. Sesamoid bones can be affected by the same spectrum of pathology as any other bone: sesamoiditis (chondromalacia) from repetitive mechanical stress, osteochondritis from injury (characterized by mottling of the sesamoid on X-ray), degenerative arthritis, inflammatory arthritis and infection.

3. Regardless of cause, the first-line treatment for sesamoid pain is to offload pressure from the first MTP joint and the sesamoids. In most instances, an insole with a plantar metatarsal pad to deflect pressure from the first metatarsal head satisfactorily achieves this. In the event of non-union of a fractured sesamoid, immobilization in a cast may be indicated. In-shoe plantar pressure measurements provide a useful means of evaluating the effectiveness of orthoses by quantifying pressure reduction (Fig. 49.3). In this case, these simple measures were sufficient to significantly ameliorate the patient's symptoms. Figure 49.3a shows Maximum Pressure Pictures of 54 Ncm^{-2} and 40 Ncm^{-2} for the right and left metatarsal heads respectively. Figure 49.3b shows the same feet, this time with an insole in the right shoe. Pressure at the metatarsal head has been reduced to 16 Ncm^{-2} on the right side, while on the left side the pressure remains high.

4. Surgical excision of part or all of one sesamoid may be considered for non-union of a fractured bone or avascular necrosis. It should be explained to the patient that relief of pain is not guaranteed. The flexor digitorum brevis tendon must be kept intact to prevent an extension deformity of the hallux.

Clinical tip: plantar pressure assessment

Plantar pressures give a good indication of foot function during gait, by quantitatively measuring the distribution of load under the foot. The example above illustrates the use

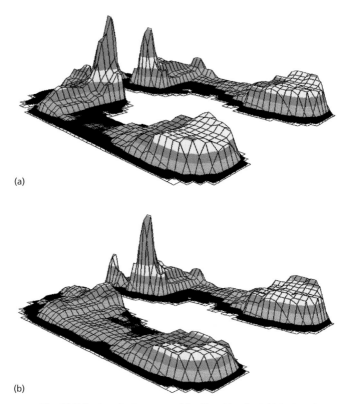

Fig. 49.3 In-shoe foot pressures (a) without insole right foot and (b) with insole right foot

of the Novel™ Pedar system. This system utilizes insoles placed within the patient's shoes. The measurement of pressures at the foot–shoe interface is the one that most resembles 'real life' walking and it also allows the analyses of a number of steps and other activities. However, the nature of the flexible insole compromises reliability compared to fixed-force platforms which provide a true vertical force measurement. Force platforms also contain more sensors, and therefore have greater resolution, but they suffer from the need for patients to 'target' the platform, which may alter normal gait.

With improving technology, plantar pressure systems are becoming more commonplace in the clinical environment. They are invaluable for the assessment of patients regarded as being at risk from high plantar pressures, particularly with diabetes and rheumatoid arthritis. Once identified as having abnormal plantar pressures, the efficacy of various therapies: footwear, orthoses, surgery, etc. can be evaluated, as in the case example above.

KEY POINTS

- True fractures of the hallux sesamoid bones are rare; they are usually stress related.
- Fracture should be differentiated from partite sesamoids.
- Sesamoid pain is treated with deflective insoles.
- Plantar foot pressure assessment is useful in assessing the effectiveness of insoles.

FURTHER READING

Orlin MN, McPoil TG (2000) Plantar pressure assessment. Physical Therapy 80:399–409.

Richardson E (1987) Injuries to the hallucal sesamoid in the athlete. Foot and Ankle International 7:229–44.

Rosenfield JS, Trepman E (2000) Treatment of sesamoid disorders with a rocker sole shoe modification. Foot and Ankle International 21(4):914–15.

Scranton P, Rutkowski R (1980) Anatomic variations in the first ray. Part II. Disorders of the sesamoids. Clinical Orthopaedics and Related Research 151:256–64.

CASE 50

A 40-year-old hill-walker presents to the clinic complaining that his ankle aches when he descends all but the flattest of slopes. New lightweight boots did not make the slightest difference to his symptoms. The radiograph is shown in Figure 50.1.

1. What is the natural history of this talar lesion?

2. How might the lesion be further assessed?

3. Is surgical treatment ever of value?

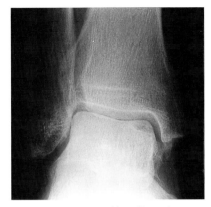

Fig. 50.1 AP ankle radiograph

Osteochondral lesions of the talus

1. Osteochondritis of the talus is generally initiated by direct trauma to the ankle. It is very similar in many respects to osteochondritis dissecans in the knee. The following radiographic classification is commonly used:

Stage I: A small area of compression of the subchondral bone. The articular cartilage remains intact.

Stage II: A partially detached osteochondral fragment. The anterior talofibular and calcaneofibular ligaments will have ruptured.

Stage III: A completely detatched fragment that remains in its talar crater.

Stage IV: A displaced fragment.

The fractures occur with a similar frequency on the medial and lateral borders of the talus. The lateral lesions are generally located in the middle third of the talar margin, as during inversion of a dorsiflexed ankle the talus rotates laterally in the frontal plane, causing impingement of its margin against the fibula. In contrast, medial lesions, caused when an inversion force is placed on a plantar flexed ankle, are sited further posteriorly at the point of impingement of the talar dome.

2. The exact nature of the lesion may be assessed by plain X-ray, tomography, CT scanning, MR imaging, or arthroscopically. Chronic lesions may develop a sclerotic margin to the bone surrounding the lesion (low intensity on T1-weighted magnetic resonance imaging).

3. Some symptomatic relief is usually gained from wearing either a medial or lateral heel flare, depending on the site of the lesion. Arthroscopic drilling should be considered for young patients with an osteochondral defect if there is only mild surrounding sclerosis of the talar bone, continuity of the cartilaginous surface and stability of the osteochondral fragment. Occasionally, it may be possible to fix a hinged fragment using small pins or screws, but once completely detached (grades III and IV), fragment removal is necessary to prevent any further abrasion of the joint surface.

KEY POINTS

- Talar osteochondritis generally follows forced ankle inversion.
- MRI is useful to determine if the fragment remains attached.
- Repair is not generally possible, although drilling of the base may be considered.
- A heel flare may be beneficial.

FURTHER READING

Berndt AL, Harty M (1959) Transchondral fractures (osteochondritis dissecans) of the talus. Journal of Bone and Joint Surgery 41-A:988–1020.

Kumai T, Takakura Y, Higashiyama I, Tamai S (1999) Arthroscopic drilling for the treatment of osteochondral lesions of the talus. Journal of Bone and Joint Surgery 81-A:1229–35.

CASE LIST

1. Aetiology of hallux rigidus
2. Freiberg's infraction
3. Hammer toe
4. Polydactyly and macrodactyly
5. Aetiology of hallux valgus
6. Plantar heel pain syndrome
7. Achilles tendon bursitis
8. Surgery of hallux rigidus
9. Metatarsalgia
10. Ganglion
11. Surgery of hallux valgus
12. Plantar fibroma
13. Venous ulceration
14. Plantar pustulosis/dermatosis
15. Fungal foot infections
16. Ingrowing toenails
17. Subungual exostosis
18. Viral warts
19. Pitted keratolysis
20. Chilblains
21. Congenital talipes equinovarus
22. Flat foot
23. Claw toe and adductus quinti digiti
24. Metatarsus adductus
25. Talocalcaneal synostosis
26. Congenital metatarsal anomalies
27. Melanoma
28. Amputation
29. Ischaemic toe
30. Chondrosarcoma of the great toe
31. Frostbite
32. Subcutaneous infection
33. Septic arthritis

Index

Note: page numbers followed by numbers in brackets indicate a question and its answer.